The Diary of Delores D'Lump

Also by Claire Laishley and published by Ginninderra Press
Did You Know We Had a Screen Door?
Writing the Wrongs of My Life

Claire Laishley

The Diary of Delores D'Lump

My Date With Breast Cancer

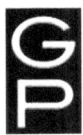

The Diary of Delores D'Lump: My Date With Breast Cancer
ISBN 978 1 74027 710 5
Copyright © Claire Laishley 2011

First published 2011
Reprinted 2015

Ginninderra Press
PO Box 3461 Port Adelaide 5015
www.ginninderrapress.com.au

Acknowledgements

Although this might be the first page you read (I say 'might' knowing I've skipped this page in books myself), it's turned out to be the last one to be written.

So here I am; I've signed off on the final edit, the publishing date is looming and I've just realised this could turn into the largest dedication ever published. You see, so many people got me to this point – the point where I can look back at this fairly dramatic time in my life and say, 'Thanks for your part in pulling me through.' But therein lays the quandary!

What happens if I forget someone? How dreadful to omit just one of the many who propped, mopped and bopped me through the journey of Delores! Yes, 'propped' me up with their strength, 'mopped' me up when it all became too much and 'bopped' with me at the pure joy of good times. My recovery is a tribute to all of you, so thanks from the bottom of my 'slightly damaged' heart. But having said that, I'll now go on to say this: there are two people I would like to mention.

Big thanks go to my publisher, Stephen Matthews at Ginninderra Press. In this literary world of constant 'Sorry, it's not right for our list' (whatever the hell that means!) Stephen has always shown faith in my writing. Thank you, man of few words – hope those two reflect my gratitude sufficiently.

And the other special mention does seem inadequate. I mean, how do you tell someone who was there for you every shitty step of the way that most of your strength came from stealing a chunk of his. HoN (Husband of Narrator), you're my hero. When a dear friend saw the ugly photo of me 'looking at the other side', she said, 'That man must really love you!' Well, believe me, it's reciprocated.

Friday 31 August

I love Fridays. Who doesn't? My three days of work are over and the weekend is just hours away. But before that, I have an entire day to clean the house, wash the clothes and do the food shopping. Sounds ordinary, I know, but I think there's still something of my mother – the 1950s housewife – in me because I love smelling the clean sheets on the bed, restocking the fridge and doing the ironing in front of Judge Judy. And this was to be another of those days. Oh, that's right... I did have a doctor's appointment mid-morning to check out a breast lump I'd discovered earlier in the week, but I wasn't particularly worried. It was very small and I'd already had two previous lumpectomies. Thankfully both lumps were benign, and the doctor did say there would probably be more over the years.

I don't know what made me put my hand up to my breast last week. I'd given up doing self-examinations since the advent of mammograms; my boobs are so lumpy (the clinical term) that I was never sure what I should be looking for. But this lump was different. It felt as though a pea had been inserted near the tip of my left nipple and, like the princess in the bed, once felt, couldn't be ignored.

My doctor has a lovely manner and a keen sense of humour. At my last visit a month earlier we had dealt with another lump, this one between my breasts, which turned out to be a sebaceous cyst. She laughed when I told her an elderly lady I know refers to them as 'herbaceous' cysts. As the doctor pierced the cyst, I told her to be careful because I might be about to sprout a bunch of parsley. And here I was showing her yet another lump.

'It doesn't look too ominous and seems disconnected,' she said, as she gently manipulated my breast. 'At least it's not pulling the nipple out of shape, so that's a good sign.' She smiled encouragement. 'Your last mammogram was only eight months ago, but just to be on the safe side, I'll send you for another one. They can do an ultrasound at the same time.' She paused. 'Can you go now?'

Bugger! I'm not going to get everything done at home today. Oh well, I guess it's better to clear this up. I nodded.

The clinic was less than a ten-minute drive from the surgery, and as I sat in the waiting room, I was struck by the number of women who had brought their partners. 'Poor things,' I thought. 'They've probably been diagnosed with cancer. I wonder how you'd cope with that.'

The couple standing at the reception desk looked to be in their early forties and were finalising their account. Each time the woman was asked a question, she turned desperate eyes to her husband. We use the term 'stunned mullet' so often, and I have sometimes wondered whether I would even recognise a mullet, let alone a 'stunned' one. In this case, however, the term did seem appropriate. And then my name was called.

The radiographer set up the machine for the mammogram and we chatted about her weekend plans.

'Just work and study, as usual,' she replied to my query.

'What about clubbing and shopping?' I thought. Had weekends changed so much from my teenage years? My maternal mantle descended as I pointed out she should allow some time for R&R, but she just smiled as she proceeded to reduce my left breast to something resembling a crêpe. Crap that hurt!

'I'll let the doctor have a look at these,' she said, waving the films in the air, 'but don't get dressed in case he needs more,' she added, disappearing through the door.

Right from the first sign I was growing breasts (and to my horror, this happened before anyone else in my class!) my breast tissue had never felt the need to confine itself to the front of my body, and had spread under my arms as well. It wasn't unusual for technicians doing the mammograms to miss getting some of this tissue on to the metal plate, so the need for extra 'shots' was fairly common. When she came back into the room, her expression told me we were not finished.

'Sorry, but the doctor needs to see a certain section a bit clearer.'

Great! Although some women sail through mammograms with little discomfort, I have always found it quite painful, and I'm convinced the reason is my lack of height. These machines are adjustable but are not geared for anyone shorter than five foot, because once the technician has laid one of 'the twins' on the plate and squeezed the bejesus out of her, they then decide she needs a ride to the ceiling!

'Right – now relax and breathe normally.' The girl's a comedian!

Then it was time for the ultrasound and this appeared to be my reward for enduring the mammogram, as the only uncomfortable part was the initial cold squirt of gel. And once the small, smooth ball was gently guided over the skin, I knew I could finally relax. It felt like a massage after a long run – not that I would really know. Oh sure, I've had massages. Still contemplating the long run, however.

This time the technician is a woman closer to my own age and we chat about everything – everything except breasts and lumps. It takes longer than I thought it would but I'm prepared to lie back and lap it up. After about ten minutes of gentle massage, she leans closer to the screen, frowns and then excuses herself. Five minutes later she returns, with a doctor in tow. They both stare at the screen and discuss what they are looking at, but the conversation is couched in medical terms, so I am none the wiser.

Then the doctor turned to me. 'It's looking a bit suspicious,' he said, 'so we'd like to take a biopsy.'

I wanted to ask how a piece of flesh could look 'apprehensive and distrustful' but realised I didn't feel like joking. I smiled – only just. 'That's fine.' My voice sounded a little higher than normal.

The doctor picked up a needle and I quickly looked away.

'I'm sorry, but once the needle is in I'll have to move it around so I can get a good sample.'

I had an insane desire to grab this doctor in his most vulnerable area and shout, 'We're not going to hurt each other, are we?' But again, I lied. 'That's fine,' I repeated.

The needle biopsy was everything he promised, and more, and I lay there trying to write a shopping list in my head. It had become so important I concentrate on any ordinary task, so I mentally trawled the aisles of my local Foodland until finally the trolley was full and the needle was withdrawn.

'I'll get the hospital pathologist to come over and have a look, and then we'll know what we're dealing with,' the doctor said. 'In the meantime, you can sit in a special waiting area we have next door.' He paused and then added, 'Or you can use the main reception area if you'd prefer.'

Why did I need a special waiting area? Was that where you waited for special news?

I turned right and headed for the general reception area, and because it was crowded, it took a few moments to locate a vacant seat. I was wedged between two much larger people, and as we had all had our personal spaces encroached upon, we focused on the incredibly loud woman on television demonstrating some sort of wonder mop. But after only a few minutes of over enthusiasm (hers not mine) I wanted out.

The 'special' area was smaller and I was the sole occupant. I grabbed a *Women's Weekly* and was surprised to find it current, but it didn't hold my interest. I was just reaching for a New Idea when the doctor walked into the room, his face squashed with concern.

'I'm going to refer you to a surgeon...Clive Hoffmann,' he said, 'I rang his rooms and he can see you this afternoon.'

For a moment I had an insane desire to laugh. You see, the surgeon shared a name with the hairdresser I went to some years ago. Perhaps this doctor standing in front of me had noticed the two stray hairs on my nipple. But surely the Venus Vibrating Razor could have coped with those!

The doctor's voice broke through my thoughts. 'He'll look after you. He did my mother-in-law's operation a few years ago.'

I bit my lower lip, as I felt an insane desire to laugh, but the doctor must have picked up on it because he allowed a small smile.

'And before you ask, yes, I do get on very well with my mother-in-law. She's more like my mother – I lost her when I was only twenty.'

The appointment was made and there was a two-hour wait. I walked outside the medical rooms and suddenly felt panic hit. A wave of nausea flowed over me and I was drenched with perspiration. This whole thing was getting out of hand. It was Friday – the day I'm supposed to be home doing washing, stripping beds and writing out shopping lists. I felt so alone, but then realised I didn't have to be. My husband answered his mobile on the third ring.

'Hi, darl, it's me,' I said, my voice a little shaky. 'Look, I didn't say anything this morning but I've been to have a breast lump checked and they don't like the look of it and I have to go and see a surgeon and I can't do this by myself.' I tripped over my words as I delivered them in a single breath.

There was a brief silence from the other end of the phone, but when he finally responded, his voice was calm. 'Right! Well, first of all, you don't have to do it by yourself – I'll be there. Now where are you?' he asked.

I told him and he talked over the logistics of how he would get to the clinic, 'I'll take a taxi, that'd be easiest – no point in having two cars there' and how soon he would get there, 'Let me just take ten minutes to finish up here.'

I wanted to scream – to tell him I didn't care about details – but one of us had to stay calm, and the chance of that person being me was not looking good.

'I'll be with you in half an hour tops – hang in there, babe,' he finished, sensing my anxiety.

I wandered down the street, glanced at my watch and was surprised to find it was already lunchtime. My stomach had been rumbling all morning, particularly during the tests, and I commented to the technician that this would probably be the only 'ultra' sound she would be able to hear. I walked into a deli, looked at the food and promptly lost my appetite.

'I should eat something,' I thought, but all I could face was a cheese and Vegemite sandwich on white bread, the same thing Mum would make me when I was unwell as a little girl. I asked for it to be toasted, but the luncheon technician took so long to actually place one piece of cheese between two pieces of Vegemite bread, I was at screaming point. I reached over the counter, grabbed the sandwich, threw some money in his direction and left the shop.

Walking back to the medical rooms, I took a bite of the sandwich and felt nauseous. I sat on the brick wall surrounding the clinic and felt cold, even though the sun was shining. Perhaps the beautiful Labrador sitting with his master a little further up the wall might like a special treat.

'Thanks, but we stick to his regular mealtimes,' his owner said. 'I don't want him to get overweight.' The man smiled an apology.

Suddenly my eyes misted and I knew I was close to tears. 'Oh no, please don't let me cry,' I thought. 'People might offer assistance and what would I say? That I need to see a surgeon and I'm scared?'

And then a taxi pulled up – my lifeline had arrived.

I held on to HoN (Husband of Narrator) so tightly that words were unnecessary. We sat in my car and I told him everything that had happened since I left home that morning. I could see him sifting things through in his mind, and while his expression remained neutral, I noticed a change in his eyes.

'It's only a small lump, thank goodness,' I said as I lifted up my T-shirt and bra and placed his finger on my nipple.

'That has to be a good sign,' he said, giving me a smile.

I don't know how we filled in the next hour, but eventually it was time for my appointment.

The surgeon was a small man with a quiet voice, and after

we sat down, he leant forward and fixed me with a direct gaze. 'Let me explain how we're going to treat your cancer,' he said.

There it was – that word – and I suddenly realised that, up to this point, I had been desperately hoping (and kidding myself) that we were merely here to organise an operation for the removal of what would turn out to be benign cyst number three.

'Just a minute,' I said, my voice having lost its usual volume. 'Are you saying the lump is definitely malignant?'

The surgeon looked stricken and leant forward. 'I'm so sorry,' he said, frowning. 'I thought you knew. I assumed you had been to your GP on the way here and it had been explained to you,' he said, concern coating his words. 'Oh dear, I am sorry.'

I managed to dig up a smile from somewhere. I wanted to assure this gentle man I was all right, that it was not his fault the situation had not been explained to me in more detail at the clinic. But at the same time I felt myself zoning out and the doctor's voice fading as the word 'cancer' gained momentum in my head.

I had sometimes wondered how you would react if you were told you had cancer. Now I didn't have to wonder any more! He waited, to gauge my reaction, but I was very busy trying to control my emotions. The last thing I wanted to do was break down and embarrass myself, and maybe everyone else. He went on to explain the operation, which he recommended I have as soon as possible, and what it would entail.

When he finished, he stood up and ushered both HoN and myself into an adjoining office, introducing us to his Breast Care Nurse. 'Claire's had a bit of a shock, Jane. She wasn't told it was cancer before she came here.'

Jane's face was awash with compassion as her arms reached out and I was engulfed in a hug. That was all I needed. The tears flowed as reality hit.

Cancer – in the breast – breast cancer. Was it all those years of smoking? Was it the years of hormone replacement therapy, the one thing that gave me back my sanity after menopause hit like a ten-ton truck? Did it matter? Oh shit, I want to run away and hide.

Sunday 2 September

We left the surgeon's rooms on Friday knowing I needed an operation – partial mastectomy, the doctor called it – but further treatment would be dependent on what he found during the operation, which was scheduled for Tuesday week. The only other appointment at this stage was for a bone scan tomorrow, Monday, and this would show if the cancer had spread anywhere else. Suddenly this whole situation seemed too enormous for just HoN and me to cope with alone – we needed the family. I don't know what I expected them to do – perhaps give me reassurance that everything would turn out all right. But how could they?

Telling my eldest son was my first priority. Daniel is in his early thirties and lives on the other side of town. We don't catch up in person a lot but stay in touch with phone and text messages. So when I rang to see if he would be home on Saturday afternoon to discuss something, he was immediately suspicious.

'What's up, Mum? Nothing serious, is it?'

'No, darling, I just want to talk to you about something – nothing to worry about.'

But when I stood in his lounge room, I had to come clean. 'Sorry, Daniel, it is a bit serious. I've been diagnosed with breast cancer.'

'I knew something was up,' he said turning, and walking quickly into the kitchen. 'How you coping, Mum?' he called out a few seconds later as he busied himself tidying the kitchen counter.

'I'm fine,' I said, pasting on a smile to prove it, as he turned and searched my face. 'At least it gives me something else to write a book about. How do you like the title My Lump is my Bitch, Yo?'

He gave a short laugh, but I could see the news had shaken him. I also knew that, being born under the sign of Leo, he would want to stay strong in front of me. We talked about general things for a while but the nonchalance was getting more difficult to maintain so I made our excuses to leave. He would also need time to digest the news quietly by himself. But as I stood at the car and wrapped my arms around my 'gentle giant', his firm hug was nearly my undoing.

Telling my younger son, Adam, was going to be more complicated. Sadly he had estranged himself from me many years earlier and, for reasons which were still not clear, wished no contact at all. This is a constant heartache in my life, and with such devastating news, I felt a desperate need to see him. But the bitterness was still there – I had to accept the situation was out of my hands.

There were two other people I needed to talk to and fortunately they lived close to Daniel. You're lucky when you find the right person to share your life with, but even luckier when a great family is part of the deal. HoN's parents, MiL (mother-in-law) and FiL (father-in-law), are the loveliest couple and have welcomed me into the family from the start. As we sat in their back garden sipping coffee and exchanging news, the strain of pretending everything was normal became too much for me.

'I'm afraid we had some bad news yesterday,' I said, horrified to hear my voice crack. It seemed very important to hold it together – to show them how well I was coping with this news, so I paused and took a deep breath. 'I've got breast cancer,' I stated, trying to keep my emotions at bay.

I knew of all the people I would share this information with, Mil would understand better than anyone. She had been diagnosed with breast cancer twenty-one years ago, and in those days, the medical support network was almost non-existent. She had spoken about going off to appointments by herself and I was in awe of the strength she displayed. She put her arms around me, and I could feel the empathy in her hug. I asked her to tell HoN's sisters and their families so we wouldn't have to go over the details again and again.

When we arrived home, there was one more person in the immediate family who needed to be informed, and that was my stepson, Brett, who is in his late teens. Although he doesn't live with us permanently, he stays regularly and, having known him since he was a toddler, I think of him as my third son. But in this instance, I felt it would be better hearing this type of news from his father.

The telephone conversation this end seemed to be going well and when HoN finished the call, I asked what Brett's reaction had been.

'He sounded OK – said he was sorry to hear the news, but he seemed all right.'

But when I looked into HoN's eyes, I saw that his emotions were close to the surface and realised that he was under an enormous strain as well. Up to this point he had been busy displaying strength for me and not allowing his true feelings to come to the surface. But speaking to his boy had almost been his undoing.

Neither HoN nor I had much of an appetite and, desperate to get a good night's sleep, I took a sleeping tablet. The last thing I needed was to lie awake going over everything in my mind. The last forty-eight hours had been emotionally exhausting and I would need my strength in the coming days.

The tablet worked well – so well that, when I opened my eyes in the morning, I felt I was fighting my way through a giant marshmallow. But Daniel's face managed to float through the white fog, and I knew I needed to hear his voice to make sure he was all right.

'I didn't say too much yesterday, Mum,' he said when he answered the phone. 'I could tell you were close to tears.'

That surprised me – I thought I had done a pretty good job of covering up my emotions.

'I'm just pleased the doc said it's treatable,' he added, his voice lighter than it was twenty-four hours ago. 'That's gotta be good, right?'

'Yes, darling, it's all good. I'll have the operation and whatever treatment I need, and it'll be sweeeet,' I said, using one of his favourite expressions.

His laugh was all I needed. We were both so busy protecting each other.

'I wish my mum was alive,' I thought. I had not felt this urgent need for my own mother in quite some time. In the last few years of her life, she had succumbed to Alzheimer's and our mother/daughter roles had been reversed. But I wanted the mother of my childhood – the one who was so strong in many ways.

I could almost hear her voice.

'We're going to get through this, darling – you know that, don't you?'

Yes, I know, Mum, but I don't think I've ever been this scared.

No, it was clear I needed to talk to someone I didn't have to be brave for.

My older brother has always been my hero in a lot of ways, and although we have lived in different states for many years, we have remained close.

'Sorry, Claire, he's away on a boy's weekend,' Janet, my sister-in-law said, 'and his mobile's out of range.' There was a pause. 'Is everything all right?' She was quick to pick up a strangeness in my voice.

'No – not really – I got some bad news on Friday. Well, it's not bad – he did say "treatable", which is good – but it's not the best news. It's been a bit of a shock – I guess no one expects to hear this.' I was talking a lot, but saying nothing. 'It's breast cancer.'

I heard her intake of breath. We are friends as well as relatives and I realised, too late, how selfish I was to tell her this news and leave her to cope with it alone over the weekend.

'It's going to be OK,' I said, putting a lift in my voice, 'it's treatable, so that's all that matters.'

We talked for a few more minutes and her questions showed her concern. Just before hanging up, she assured me that 'Bruff' would get the news as soon as she could reach him. I hoped that wasn't going to be too long.

Monday 3 September

I was exhausted before the day had even started – emotion does that to me. I can knock myself out physically and never feel the bone-aching weariness which comes from having my emotions hung out to dry. And speaking of bones, I had an appointment at the hospital for a bone scan this morning. This is a test to detect abnormalities in bones and soft tissue, and will indicate whether the cancer has travelled to other parts of my body.

As I sat in the large waiting room of the hospital, I tried not to think about the ramifications if the cancer was found in other areas of my body. HoN sat beside me and as I glanced around I noticed, not only other husbands and wives, but a mother and daughter and even a grandfather with his grandson. This was a human Noah's Ark – everyone came in pairs – although there was one man sitting by himself. But just as I was wondering where his support crew was, a woman walked into the waiting room from the direction of the doctor's office. The husband looked at his wife expectantly, but she shook her head.

'I won't know for three days,' she whispered, and he reached for her hand.

I wondered if my eyes had the same fear reflected in them.

I concentrated on a print on the wall with the caption 'Sunshine over the Olgas' by Vicence Selak. I repeated the artist's name over and over in my mind. 'Is it pronounced Vichensay or Vikense,' I wondered, 'or maybe just plain Vincent or Vi-sen-say?'

I was too scared to stop concentrating in case I realised why I was sitting there. And then it was my turn. The nurse showed me into a cubicle, handed me a paper gown and told me to remove most of my clothes. My eyes strayed to a notice on the wall.

'Place gown in bin in passage after use or you may take them home. They are good for washing windows, painting smocks or washing the dog.'

As I loathe washing windows, am not in the habit of painting anything (and that includes smocks) and fail to see how a flimsy piece of paper could protect you from a dog hell-bent on ridding its fur of a wading pool of water, my gown was destined for the bin.

The nurse then led me into a small room where I was injected with a radioactive tracer which is absorbed into the bones. I had an insane desire to ask the staff if they could turn the lights off to see if I glowed in the dark, but thought I was probably better off not knowing. Maybe it was so I couldn't run away from treatment – that no matter where I was, my glow would show!

As it was going to take a while for the substance to travel through my body, we were told to come back in three hours, so HoN suggested lunch. We wandered down to the local shopping precinct which boasted many quality restaurants and I was quite surprised to find I had an appetite. We sat over large bowls of pasta and even larger glasses of wine talking about the trivia which makes up a lot of the conversation between husbands and wives. We talked about everything, but studiously avoided the topic which started with the words 'what if'. And too soon it was time to return to the hospital for the scan.

This part of the procedure took another hour, and involved lying still on a cold metal platform as the gamma camera hovered over my body and took various images. My eyes strayed to the only bit of colour in the room which was a poster divided into twelve squares. This one carried the caption 'Frogs and Flora'.

'Not a lot of thought put in here,' I decided, as each square displayed an example of either a frog or, you guessed it, a flora. I couldn't help wondering who on earth decided this was what patients needed to look at while an enormous machine hovered over them trying to pick up rogue cancer cells. My mind escaped into some of our favourite holidays for the next fifty or so minutes, but when that ceased to distract me, my eyes strayed back to the poster.

The frog in the top right-hand corner was a grumpy-looking bastard and, with his wide girth and poxy-looking skin, reminded me of a hairdresser I once knew in Melbourne. I christen thee, Arturo the Amphibian! The one sitting in the box directly underneath wasn't much prettier, and although I thought I could detect a twinkle in his eyes, Turdis the Toad seemed to fit him well.

I had just moved on to the tiny black one in the bottom left-hand corner of the poster, who still had the innocence of youth, so I named him Timothy Tadpole, when the technician was telling me the scan was finished and I could get dressed and sit back in the waiting room.

Ten minutes later, HoN and I were sitting in front of the doctor.

'It'll be three days before the results come through,' he said. I was not surprised, but how could I make that time pass quickly?

Tuesday 11 September

As it turned out, those three days of waiting for the bone scan results passed surprisingly fast. Two of the days I was busy at my part-time job doing administration work for my cousin's interior decorating business and the other day was spent volunteering at the RSPCA.

It feels like months since the diagnosis but it's only been eleven days. I'm still fairly numb, going through the motions of everyday stuff, but nothing is sinking in too deeply, except one very important fact: there was no cancer found anywhere else.

When I received the results of the bone scan last week, I felt as if all the energy was leaving my body. Like a balloon deflating, the tension I had built up seemed to ooze from every pore, leaving me feeling like a rag doll, but in a state of euphoria. Unfortunately the euphoria didn't last very long.

Daytime is fine – well, relatively fine – but I dread the nights. I sit up in bed reading until I'm so tired my whole body is aching and crying out for sleep. But the minute I put the book down and switch off the bedside lamp, my brain goes into overdrive.

'Cancer is a word, not a sentence,' echoes over and over again in my head. How often that phrase is used, but suddenly, it was personal. Cancer may be a word, but it's a bloody terrifying one from where I'm viewing it.

As soon as I opened my eyes this morning I was hit by the silence – the kind of silence which only comes in the middle of the night. I glanced across at the clock; two-forty a.m. Oh yes, I remember now. It's today I go to hospital for a partial mastectomy or, as I call it, half a boob job.

Since puberty, I've hated my breasts, even though some of my flat-chested friends said they envied me. As far as I was concerned, they could have them! I joked with one friend about booking in to hospital for a double operation, where my surgeon performs a reduction on me and passes over the excess to her surgeon.

I wandered downstairs and joined my beautiful silver tabby cat on the couch. She welcomed the company and rearranged her body to fit with mine. I smiled as I remembered the phone call from my son, Daniel, yesterday, to say he'd be thinking of me when I go in for the operation. I immediately felt guilty – only because the previous day I had wondered if he would remember. Oh, ye of little faith!

I picked up the book I'm reading at present, a James Patterson called *Suzanne's Diary to Nicholas*. Not his usual style, but I've lost myself in the story, which is exactly what I need. When I slipped back in to bed a couple of hours later and snuggled up to HoN, he opened his eyes and looked deeply into mine.

'How are you feeling, babe?' he said, cupping my face in his hand.

'Scared,' I stuttered, and when the tears started I was afraid they would never stop.

He just held me tightly and I was grateful for his understanding silence.

We were due at the hospital early, and HoN sensed my increasing tension.

As we walked across the foyer toward the reception area, he suddenly stopped and grinned. 'OK, I'll come clean. I hate broad beans and I do look at other women!'

I frowned and he pointed to a sign above his head. It read 'Admissions'. I collapsed with laughter and felt the tension dissipate.

The hospital is small and modern, set in immaculately cared for grounds, and I pretended I was checking in to a five-star hotel. It didn't take too much imagination either as we were ushered into a private room, given a complimentary newspaper and a dinner menu, which even included a wine list. My eyes travelled to the almost obligatory nature print on the wall (this one unnamed) but it had the regulation blue/purple river meandering through fields of green and yellow with the standard fluffy cloud in Delft-blue sky – a scene apparently geared to engender calm in the patient. Memo to decorator: it doesn't bloody well work!

There was a purple pinboard on the wall opposite the bed, so you would have somewhere to display your Get Well cards, and the black-headed tacks to affix the cards to the board had been made into a smiley face. But what happened if you didn't get any cards? Did they remove the board so you wouldn't get a complex? Note to self: phone MiL, who saves everything, and ask her to bring in a stack of used get well cards, just in case!

I had only just changed and settled myself in bed when the 'affable anaesthetist' bounced into the room, gave me a broad smile and introduced himself. He was probably just one of those happy people who loved life, but I couldn't help wondering if maybe he had pinched a bit of his own medication.

After he left, I glanced at HoN, who was sitting on the end of the bed. I wanted to tell him to go off to work, go for a walk or just go and do whatever he wanted – but I couldn't. I was too selfish. He was my lifeline. While he was there, I had to hold it together. We managed to fill in the next couple of hours talking and glancing at the television until a male orderly arrived to wheel me down the corridor to surgery.

'Nice touch,' he said, smiling at the tiara perched on my head.

I felt an explanation was necessary. 'When I told my interstate friend about my diagnosis, she sent me a care package full of thoughtful gifts to lift my spirits. This,' I said, tapping the tiara, 'was sitting on top.'

I looked up at the orderly's face, and even from my upside-down angle lying on the trolley, I could see his smile.

'She also felt it important my lump had a name – something foreign and exotic – and she decided to call it Delores.

By this time, we had arrived at the ritzy little theatre booked for this event, and our master of ceremonies was waiting inside. He also smiled behind his carnivale mask, as his eyes strayed to the crown jewels on my head.

'I'm so glad you could all make it to Delores's coming out party,' I said to the other assembled 'guests'.

It was a pity about the rather uninteresting ball gown I'd been given – a pale blue smock I wasn't even allowed to do up. At least I had my bling. But as the drip was inserted and my head tripped the light fantastic, the furthest thought from my mind was 'Let's party'!

It only seemed like two minutes later when I woke in recovery feeling lightheaded. The nurse asked how I felt and I replied 'Terrific', as I listened to the woman next to me dry-reach, groan and dry-reach again. Then the orderly was wheeling me back into my room and MGM (my gorgeous man) was waiting with an armful of flowers.

'I wonder what time dinner is,' I said to HoN, and he looked doubtful, but I was already anticipating the roast beef, chocolate mousse and glass of wine I had ordered earlier. But no sooner did I start eating than the nausea rose up, and HoN had to take over – the meal, not the nausea – and as soon as he finished, I ordered him home. It had been an exhausting day for both of us, and my final thought before I gave in to the leftover anaesthetic was 'Thank God that's over.'

Saturday 15 September

I was only in hospital overnight Tuesday. I felt so good when I woke up Wednesday morning, and must have looked all right, as I was given the all clear to head home. But then a phone call on Thursday from the surgeon stopped me in my tracks.

'I'm sorry,' he said. 'We've found grade 2 cancer in one of the lymph nodes we took on Tuesday. Unfortunately we'll have to go back in and take a larger sample to make sure the cancer hasn't gone any further.'

He went on to explain he had organised the operation for the next day, Friday, and mentioned it would be a larger operation than the first as I needed a drip inserted for a few days and they like to keep you in until the drip is removed. He muttered something about 'clusters', but I was rapidly tuning out.

On the way to the hospital on Friday afternoon, we stopped at the local newsagent to buy some magazines and my hand reached out to a stuffed bear with a cute face, sitting on the counter. Whether it was the memory of my beloved teddy that I would never let out of my sight when I was little, I don't know, but I decided this bear needed to come with me to hospital.

I was given the same room I had vacated a few days earlier and the staff greeted me warmly. And when I was wheeled into theatre mid-afternoon, Dr Clive was there once again, and I remembered part of the conversation we had about the need for a second operation, and how little I said at the time.

'Well, if it isn't Sir Clive of Clusters,' I said, and grinned. 'Ready to do battle with Dymphna Lymph and the Nodes?'

I was rewarded with a smile.

'I was wondering if you would like me to tidy up the excess skin on the side of your breast,' Sir Clive asked, and I suppressed a smile at his delicate explanation. I have often commented to the nurses responsible for my mammograms that I have enough breast tissue under both arms to warrant a four-cup bra (should such an animal exist).

I nodded. 'That'd be great…thanks.'

Just before I headed off with the fairies, I had a vision of my new left boob; with the reduction in size and the 'excess' tidied up, this could well become the template for 'two trimmed tits down the track'. But this time, when I came out of the anaesthetic, I felt sore and a wave of depression washed over me.

'I hope they've got it all this time,' I thought, 'because I'm not going through this again.'

I turned my head and caught sight of the small brown bear we had bought that morning sitting on the chest of drawers next to the bed. I suddenly knew what I would call him. 'Muchcan,' I said out loud, to see how it sounded. Perfect – short for 'How much can Claire Bear?'

The nurse called by and gave me a tablet for the nausea and I managed to sleep through most of the night, but when I woke this morning, I was instantly aware of the soreness in my left breast. The area around the drip was tender and the wound had been oozing overnight, so I decided to have a shower. As I stood in the cubicle with the plastic drain bag filled with a watery bloody substance hooked over my arm, I felt like a vampire going off to the ball complete with mid-evening refreshments in my Dracula's dilly bag. I turned my face up to the stream of water and tried to let the water wash off the negativity which seemed to be sticking to me as strongly as the adhesive from the pressure bandage.

After the shower, I grabbed a clean hospital gown but then tossed it to one side. I decided these unflattering garments made you look sick, even if you felt all right. Instead I opted for a pair of white satin pyjamas I had bought especially for the occasion.

I have always loved the fashions of the 1930s and 1940s, and white satin lounging pyjamas worked so well for Jean Harlow – why not me! And the new white gown to go on top. Didn't they call them theatre coats in Harlow's days? How appropriate – even though I was wearing my coat after my theatre visit. But when I moved to the mirror a few minutes later to brush my hair, I noticed a growing red stain on the left side of my pyjama top and realised my wound was still bleeding.

Just then, the day shift nurse walked in. 'How are you feeling, Claire?' she asked.

I sat down on the bed, opened my mouth to respond and burst into tears.

She sat down next to me and reached for my hand. 'You know, I was going to call my daughter Claire,' she said, as she smiled and stroked my hand. 'That was until I saw her. She looked more like a Charli than a Claire.'

I wiped my eyes and managed a smile as she went on to explain.

'You see, to me a Claire has to be refined and elegant, and my girl looked a bit of a tomboy.'

I could understand what she meant. I was certainly doing 'refined and elegant' so well this morning!

The rest of the day was taken up with relatives and friends calling in, and I managed to keep the depression at bay. But after dinner, when everything was quiet and the nursing staff were busy with an emergency at the other end of the floor, I had time to think.

Being in hospital conjured up opposing emotions for me; on one hand it felt slightly claustrophobic and I had an almost desperate need for some fresh air, but no sooner had that thought entered my head, I was also wrapped in an overwhelming feeling of safety – safe within these four walls – and I was reluctant to venture into the world ever again.

Life in hospital was so simple. It revolved around incidental things, like how many millilitres of fluid had I built up in my drain, which pain relief did I require this hour (my favourite was a little Aussie number in green and gold), which nurse would be coming on for the next shift and what time was the food trolley arriving.

Just as I was pondering the last question, my mobile registered a text message. My dear friend interstate, the one who named Delores, had somehow picked up on my depression and was intent on boosting my spirits.

> Hve jst tkn u round gorgeous markt pretending we were tog. U chose yummy jacket w matching scarf 4 me so I bought it. True!! Then we sat on grass – laughed and sipped latte – full fat and all. Then ate trendy wraps w tasty dips and charcoal lamb. Sadly u over there in silk pjs. I willing the days away when normality will rtrn. Wish I cud pop in 4 visiting hrs and show off my jacket u made me buy love u lots xxx

How could I stay down with friends like this?
I replied immediately.

> Am sure jkt is gorgeous – u put smile on my face, lovely girl. Wud giv eye teeth 4 decent coffee stead of brown dust served here. Lotsaluv

She still senses depression, so decides to give me something else to think about.

> Can u help friend out. Rcvd wedding invite and dress code is 'morning suit' – lunch on river bank nr ski fields. Wot in hell I wear?

My depression lifts as the creative juices flow.

> Being on rvr bnk u cud wr straw hat n parasol but with ski flds near u nd parka n piste xpreshun. bugger it – jst wr something black n tell her yr invite said 'mourning' suit xx

Sometimes it's just the smallest things which have the largest effect. There's a very good reason we handpick our friendships. Through a text gossip session, I was able to drag things back in perspective. Did I thank you enough, dear Lizzie?

Monday 17 September

It's been a strange day. I'm still in hospital as my drain hasn't been removed yet. I woke very early – could have been the patients' bells ringing or perhaps nervousness about receiving the test results later today. My surgeon, Sir Clive of Clusters, explained he needed to test the tissue taken from around the affected lymph node to ensure the outside edges were clear of cancer. I was finding it hard to imagine how a lump the size of a pea could have done so much damage already. Surely it hadn't had time to travel further?

I actually prayed this morning. It was the first time in many, many years and it's amazing how we remember our faith when we need something! Religion was an important but fairly subtle part of my younger years. My paternal grandfather was a dour Methodist gentleman who put the fear of God into me on the rare occasions when we visited. My father, however, enjoyed his religion, taking Sunday school classes and organising church concerts, and both he and my mother belonged to the choir. My brother and I were part of several church youth groups and these provided a great social life when we were young.

So here I was closing my eyes and conjuring up the image of Jesus – the one taught to me at Sunday school – with those all knowing eyes, a beautiful blue halo and the soft hands with long fingers brought together in prayer. The first thing I felt I should do was to beg this higher power for forgiveness for deserting him. I tried to think up excuses and then laughed. Who was I kidding? He'd see straight through me! Then I made promises I hoped I could keep, if only he would take away any remaining cancer.

I left my breakfast untouched and couldn't even face morning tea as my stomach churned and the hours ticked by. But then the doctor with the quiet demeanour, gentle smile and direct gaze was standing at the end of my bed.

'The test results have shown no further cancer in the tissue that was taken.' His smile widened slightly.

Once more my body collapsed in on itself and a large sigh was dragged from the depths of my stomach. He waited a few moments while I soaked in the good news. But I was only one patient on his rounds this morning and there were other things he needed me to be aware of.

'You're going to need a lot of rest so you can deal with the emotional strain of, not only your reactions, but other people's as well,' he said, fixing me with his direct gaze. 'And there's the possibility of lymphodoema – ten per cent of patients suffer from it.'

I offered a strained smile. 'They're pretty good odds, aren't they?' I said, begging him to agree.

'You'd be better off with zero per cent,' he replied. Was that a flash of sympathy across his face at my naivety? He mentioned a follow-up appointment in a few days to talk further treatment and, with a gentle smile, he left the room.

I was just reaching for my mobile to tell HoN the good news when the male nurse on duty came rushing in.

'I've just heard the news,' he said, 'and I'm so happy for you, Claire – that's really, really great.'

This guy had turned in to my new best friend as soon as I came in to hospital. No, really. Think about it. How many blokes would you stand in front of naked except for a pair of Bridget Jones's knickers whilst discussing your favourite movies? So his reaction to my news was very special.

Ten minutes later I was still grinning when Jane the breast care nurse arrived, and I shared the news with her. She wrapped me in a warm hug and told me how thrilled she was, then handed me a purple satin cushion in the shape of a crescent moon with a strap attached. I looked puzzled so she hooked the strap over my left shoulder, settled the cushion next to my breast and gently rested my arm against the padding. As the pressure from my arm was taken away from my tender breast, the relief was instantaneous, and I knew this design must have originated from a fellow sufferer. But then it was down to business. Jane carefully outlined the things I would now have to be aware of. There would be daily exercises to alleviate the numbness in the armpit. Extra care would have to be taken when travelling on long flights. I must always wear gloves to garden and wash dishes. I must make sure doctors and nurses used my right arm only for injections and taking blood pressure. She explained about lymphodoema and the side effects.

That dreaded word again – lymphodoema – and all I heard was 'swollen arm'. When I was about nine years old, a girlfriend's mother had a mastectomy and all I could remember was her one normal-size arm, while the other was enormous. Whenever I was in the same room with her, I couldn't take my eyes off it. Now here I was facing the possibility of having the same thing happen to me.

Jane's voice suddenly dragged me back to the present. 'Watch for lines travelling down the arm, Claire – not a good sign,' she said. It means that fluid is building up and, if this happens, it will have to be removed with a syringe.

'Hell's teeth,' I thought, 'the cancer may not have travelled anywhere else but the damage it's already done is really starting to impact.'

'Stop!' There was a scream echoing in my head. 'This is too much information. I want time to savour the good news.'

But Jane was unaware of the inner turmoil I was experiencing because I smiled and pretended I was taking all this information on board. She mentioned again how thrilled she was at the good news, and I knew she would be distraught if she knew how upset I was. Or maybe she'd dealt with so many patients, there was no standard reaction.

These BCNs (breast care nurses) are a great idea and we were really lucky to find our particular Boobs, Chests and Norks girl. From the minute I met her, I felt her compassion and suspected she would become very important over the coming months.

Jane impressed upon me right from the beginning, she was on call at any time. 'I've had phone calls in the middle of the night and while I was supermarket shopping, but it doesn't matter, Claire. If you need me, I'm there for you.'

As soon as she left, I phoned HoN and told him the cancer had not been found anywhere else.

His voice carried his excitement. 'That's the best news I could hear, babe,' he said. 'I bet you're relieved.'

I said I was, but I don't think he was convinced.

'How about I come to the hospital a bit earlier today?'

I grunted my relief as I realised how exhausted I was. Once again the emotions had drained me mentally and physically. But I was also experiencing panic – wanting to crawl away and hide. What was wrong with me? Everyone seemed happy except me. I had just heard the best news ever but it was not bringing me the joy it should have.

I fell asleep waiting for HoN and when I woke he was by my bed smiling down at me. I started babbling – trying to tell him how I was feeling – but I couldn't seem to put it into words.

He frowned. 'Yes, but it couldn't be a better outcome, could it? You've got to be happy with that,' he said.

I nodded and realised the emotions I was experiencing could not be explained, even to the person I felt closest to. He asked what else the doctor had said on his visit and I tried to remember the details. He questioned me several times on some minor point, and that was all I needed. Suddenly the floodgates opened and I was crying. And this was no quiet sniff into a tissue – no way! These were gut-wrenching sobs that seemed to come from deep within and took much more effort to bring to the surface. They were the sort of tears that transform your face into a wet, twisted sneaker that's lost any visible means of support, and also turns your eyes into large, fleshy slits.

HoN was contrite, hugging me and saying how sorry he was, but I could tell he was confused, the poor darling. He had been under enormous strain as well and I was just beginning to realise it.

When you are diagnosed with a serious illness, you're surrounded by supportive medical staff, and you are extremely lucky if you have family and friends to lean on. All the attention is on the patient, but often, standing quietly next to you is a partner who is going through the hell of watching someone they love trying to cope with their illness. The patient is allowed, and often expected, to ride a roller coaster of emotions, but the support crew often feel they mustn't give in – it's their role to be strong.

How could I do this to him – the man who had been so supportive and strong? And that thought made me cry even harder!

Friday 21 September

I had an appointment with the surgeon, Sir Clive of Clusters, today to discuss further treatment. He was running late and we had over an hour's wait – time for me to flip through every magazine in the waiting room and read absolutely nothing. As soon as we sat down in his office, he started talking about my particular cancer and presented us with a sheet of graphs. My eyes skimmed the page but I could feel myself drowning in percentages. HoN, however, had pulled his chair closer to the desk and was riveted to the document. As he has an analytical mind, the doctor was speaking his language.

'So everything looks good until we come to here,' the doctor said, pointing to the last line. 'This shows the cancer is HER2 positive, and that's why I'm going to recommend a compilation treatment of chemotherapy, radiotherapy, hormone treatment and a drug called Herceptin.'

The doctor's words somehow penetrated the fog of my brain, but I couldn't speak. Only one word ricocheted around my head – chemotherapy – and the picture this word evoked. No hair, no eyebrows, no eyelashes. No way! But then I remembered a woman I worked with some years ago who had breast cancer and needed chemotherapy. She had worn some sort of hat filled with ice during her treatments and retained her hair. Yes, I'll have one of those, I thought. But what about my brows and lashes? Would I have to wear six small ice strips to stop the same thing happening to them?

I was suddenly dragged back to the present when I heard HoN ask what the percentages of survival were if I undertook all this treatment, and Sir Clive's response with more statistics.

'Those odds are good, babe,' HoN said, trying to gauge my reaction. 'It's really quite positive.'

He had probably noticed I was not contributing much to the conversation, and I still didn't – just nodded. Yes, I already felt positive – positively depressed! But I couldn't voice this out loud. HoN was so desperate to find something good in all of this information.

It was quiet in the car on the way home, both of us busy with our own thoughts. HoN needed his statistics and figures to make sense of all this – I just operated on the emotional level. The only thing which was certain at this stage was the long treatment regime which stretched ahead. My plans for being healthy and over all this by Christmas had just taken a nosedive. But as soon as we walked in the door, we started to discuss what the doctor had said, and I was stunned when HoN made the following statement.

'I've been thinking about it, and if it was my body, I wouldn't have the chemotherapy,' he said, watching my reaction closely.

Initially I was shocked he would even think about going against the doctor's suggestion. But then I thought about it and realised I actually had a choice. I didn't have to have any treatment if I didn't want it. The doctors could only recommend, but the final decision was mine.

What do I do? What happens if I don't have it? And what will happen to my body if I fill it with 'a toxic tequila' of chemotherapy drugs? I could feel the start of a panic attack and I lashed out verbally.

'Well, it's not your body, and it's my decision to make,' I snapped, and immediately regretted it when I saw HoN's face cloud with emotion 'Oh shit, darling, I'm so sorry – I know you're only trying to help.'

We hugged and he accepted my apology with a smile, but because we were both trying to deal with completely separate emotions, discussion seemed pointless. We soon drifted off to separate rooms where we could be alone with our thoughts. Later that night we were watching television, still keeping our thoughts to ourselves, when HoN switched the sound down and turned towards me.

'I've been thinking quite a bit about the chemotherapy,' he said, 'and I've had a change of heart. I'd have it, if I was you.'

I told him it wasn't necessary to agree with me just so we were on the same page, but knew his natural honesty wouldn't allow this anyway. He explained he had been looking at the percentages in a different way, the opposite to the way he first approached them. Instead of saying that having chemotherapy increases my chances of living past ten years by only five per cent, he had now 'extrapolated' (or whatever the hell these financial people do) and could see that, without chemotherapy, one person in twenty could be affected by a recurrence of cancer.

I felt at peace knowing he had reached this conclusion through rationale, and not the need to agree with me, because over the last few hours, I had pretty much decided to go ahead with the chemotherapy treatments anyway. You see, the thing which frightened me more than losing my hair for a few months was the chance the cancer would come back if I didn't do everything I could to get rid of it now.

I didn't want to go to bed with the thought of chemo treatment hanging over my head (or hair!) so decided to think about something else. I was not familiar with the drug Herceptin, which had been recommended in the compilation treatment and, as you do, decided to Google it.

I hadn't really paid attention in the doctor's room and felt more comfortable taking in the information at my own pace. But I wasn't too thrilled to read that one of the side effects of this particular drug was a small chance of heart failure. As I turned out the light and pulled up the covers, my final thoughts revolved round our family history of heart problems. Perhaps I had better do a bit more research before I agree to that particular stage of treatment.

Thursday 27 September

Time to meet my oncologist – one doctor I hoped I would never have to put a possessive pronoun in front of. But having said that, HoN and I took to this doctor immediately. With a first name of Tabitha, I was desperately hoping she could weave some sort of magic for me, but her agreement with Sir Clive about the necessity for the compilation treatment just confirmed once again the long road to recovery. Not only did she agree with the treatment recommended but the reasons for her decisions were explained to us so the statistical side (for HoN) and the emotional side (for me) were addressed.

'With everything considered, it's probably going to be about twelve months of treatment,' she said, as she left the room to fetch some brochures.

I sat listening as the picture got bleaker, and this final statement confirmed my worst thoughts. The long arduous road to recovery was stretching further and further into the distance. But when I mentioned this to HoN, he tried to break it down.

'Yes, but the intensive side is only until next April – if you think of it like that, it will be easier.'

Poor darling! Again he was grappling for positives and all I could do was concentrate on the negatives. In the end it didn't really matter how I thought of it. With the ongoing Herceptin treatment, I'd still be reminded I had cancer until Christmas of the following year – another fifteen months!

A few minutes later the doctor returned and started to explain the side effects of chemotherapy. 'Apart from hair loss, which is pretty much a given with the particular drugs you'll be taking, one of the other side effects of chemo is a certain vagueness, so be prepared for that,' my WWW (Wonderful Wicked Witch) said.

'And how will I know it's the chemo?' HoN asked, and I was pleased to realise the doctor had a sense of humour when she laughed.

Then there was a knock on the door, and we were introduced to Sophie, the clinical nurse.

Tabitha explained that Sophie would be supervising a lot of my chemo sessions and I looked at this slightly built pretty brunette with the large, brown doe-like eyes and knew I had reached 'that' age. You know the age – when you look at figures of authority and think, 'But you're soooo young.'

'Sophie will become very important to you both over the coming months,' WWW said, interrupting my thought.

'Why? Do you do ironing, Sophie?' HoN asked.

Sophie laughed, and I knew we'd get on.

As we walked back to the car, I mentioned again how nervous I was about the inevitable hair loss, so HoN suggested we go wig shopping. Through experience, he knew the sooner any problem I had was addressed, the better I could handle a situation. After a quick lunch, we headed for a wig shop in the city the doctor had recommended.

I sat in front of a mirror as the assistant placed different styles of wigs on my head, and my heart plummeted. 'I look like my mother in the throes of dementia when she forgot to do her hair!' I stated, petulantly.

'You can have them trimmed,' the assistant quickly added, 'Sometimes they are a bit full.'

'Don't know about full,' I thought. 'I'd have to be as pissed as a fart to walk down the street with this thing on my head.'

The persistent assistant seemed determined the day would not be wasted – for her at least – so as quickly as I pulled one hirsute hat from my head and chucked it on the table in front of me, she was poised with a smile and a replacement.

Possibly nothing would have looked good on me that day as the face peering from under the fulsome fringes was decidedly ugly. The forehead had collapsed into a corrugation of frown lines, the eyes were not only swimmingly moist but tinged with red streaks and both sides of the mouth arrowed towards the floor.

In a last-ditch attempt to try and make this thing work, I pointed to a wig on the top shelf. It had been styled in the shape of a bob, reminiscent of the way I wore my hair in the 1960s. I had always loved that style. I held the front of the wig firm as the assistant pulled it over my head. After a couple of tugs, a bit of a flick and a swish of the fringe, she stood back and smiled at my reflection.

I stared at the face in the mirror, but couldn't even recognise myself. No, that's not quite correct. I recognised myself all right. A child of the 60s trying to recapture her lost youth. Mutton. Lamb. Shriek! My eyes filled with tears.

'Sorry, I just can't do this any more,' I said, pulling the wig off and sending a desperate look in HoN's direction. 'I want to go home.'

As we walked out of the shop and headed down the arcade, the tears were close to spilling over.

HoN turned to me. 'All right, I agree – maybe a wig isn't the answer for you. But I think it's important you have a plan about how you'll cope with the hair loss before it happens. Let's look at scarves and turbans. Didn't the doctor say they have a good selection at the hair salon attached to the hospital down the road?'

My flight response was going into overdrive – I just wanted to get away from all this reality. But I also knew my man didn't want me going home with such a negative attitude and, because he was trying so hard to support me, I felt I owed him this.

The selection of hats and turbans in the hair salon attached to the hospital was huge and I was surprised how smart they all looked. As I placed a turban on my head, I could feel my spirits lifting. I grabbed one of the scarves and wound it around the turban, and suddenly the prospect of losing my hair was not as frightening as I had imagined.

We walked out of the salon fifteen minutes later with the makings of a 'new me' clutched in a brown paper bag. HoN, you're a bloody genius!

Sunday 30 September

It was the Australian Football League Grand Final yesterday – Port Power vs Geelong. Not that I really cared. When I moved to Adelaide from Melbourne in my late teens, I had vowed to give up that particular religion, and had only taken a minor interest in the sport since then. But I couldn't help being aware of the impact this one day in September had on most of the population as I wandered around a near-deserted shopping mall at two-thirty in the afternoon. The lack of shoppers suited me just fine because I was on a mission.

Now I had accepted that hair loss was inevitable, and a cover-up solution had been decided upon, I was prepared to throw my all into getting organised before even one hair fell out. I thought there would be more choice at one of the two large department stores in the complex so that is where I headed, and a middle-aged shop assistant was only too pleased to join me in the exercise when I explained why I was buying scarves by the armful.

'You have a wonderful attitude to all this,' she said, leaning forward and wrapping me in a warm hug. 'You're an inspiration.'

I felt so guilty. She wouldn't have made that statement had she witnessed my petulance in the wig shop on Friday!

At one shop, the owner even offered me a discount, which I was only too pleased to accept. I had already figured out that whatever I saved over the next few months on shampoo, conditioner, cuts and colour, I was rapidly spending on large pieces of colourful silk.

Satisfied with my purchases, I was heading back to the car when I walked past a shop which I usually ignored. From the doof doof beat of music and the minuscule tops in the window, this shop screamed 'under 20s' and therefore held no interest for me. But my attention was caught by a display of headwear on a table just inside the door.

There were fascinating fascinators all fluff and feathers, and hippy headbands reminiscent of the 1970s, but something else had caught my eye. At the front of the table was the head of a store dummy sporting an elegant turban with a jewelled brooch in the centre. Just as I picked up the turban to try it on, a young shop assistant walked over.

'You right, there?' she asked.

'I was just admiring this – isn't it gorgeous?'

'Yeah, I loved it when I first saw it,' she said, 'but then I tried it on like, and I looked like one of those chronic chemo women who've lost their hair!' Her eyes widened, the eyebrows shot up and her right nostril followed.

I am usually quite outspoken when comments are made that I disagree with, but in this instance, I was lost for words. Perhaps she was so young she had never been personally affected by cancer through friends or family. But with the statistics of one person in eight getting breast cancer, she wouldn't remain untouched for much longer.

I suddenly lost all interest in shopping. I dropped the turban on the table, walked out of the shop and headed to the car park.

Was that going to be me – a 'chronic chemo woman'? Is that how people would think of me? But as I drove home, my sensitivity started to turn to anger and I began to formulate the response I would love to deliver in a few week's time when the chemotherapy drugs had taken away my hair.

With a turban and scarf covering my baldness, I would walk into the shop and look her in the eye. 'Hello. Remember me? No, you probably don't – I wasn't one of those chronic chemo people when we first spoke!'

The rest of the day, however, had been a success, and I had to admit I had probably gone a bit overboard with the number of scarves I purchased.

Suffice to say, HcN took one look at the assortment which

almost covered the entire queen size bed, and made a decision. 'I think you need a hat stand for this lot,' he said.

We started at Freedom and finally found the perfect one at Harvey Norman's. Well, perfect in my eyes, that is – right colour, right shape. Only thing was, it came in a flat pack! Now this is what I class as a sign of true love, as the last time a piece of furniture came in pieces, the air was turned a paler shade of blue as HoN attempted to fit part A into part B.

When we arrived home, I studiously ignored the box on the lounge room floor until I experienced a fit of conscience. After all, this hat stand was going to make my life easier – I really should show my appreciation and put it together myself. But after I had made sure there were 20 x F1 screws, 8 x F2 screws and 4 little rubber thingos, I was exhausted and felt I'd done enough.

I guess HoN will live to regret the next four words he uttered for a long time. And even if he didn't, he'll think even more carefully before he speaks in the future.

'Need a hand, babe?' he called, from his supine position on the couch.

Let the fun begin!

Thursday 4 October

At last the stitches are out! The doctor was going to remove them a fortnight ago but the wound hadn't healed enough. It's been quite uncomfortable and very tender, but the half-moon satin cushion that Jane, my BCN (boobs, chests and norks) gal gave me in the hospital has been a godsend, and I don't travel too far these days without Priscilla the Purple Pilla.

I should have felt more excited this morning when we drove to the doctor's rooms – after all, this was one more step back to normalcy – but a feeling of dread swamped any euphoria I may have felt. At the first attempt to remove the stitches, the surgical tape had clung to my skin with an iron grip, and the whole procedure became a form of torture.

Five minutes into the exercise I was prepared to admit to anything they wanted to hear, if only they would just stop the pain. Yes, all right, my feet did touch the bottom of the pool during my swimming certificate for freestyle back in 1956. And it was me who took money from your purse for lollies, Mum – twice. And – if it'll help – I am running a drug operation (albeit a small one) from my downstairs toilet. OK, the last one's a bit of a stretch, but hey, I'll admit to anything. Just promise not to hurt me.

So, as some liquid was rubbed over the bandage and fingers grabbed the edge, I gritted my teeth and tried to think of something pleasant. Fiji, crystal clear waters, white sands, tropical breeze – ohm – ohm – OUCH! And then it was over, just like that.

I was so busy thanking the doctor and the nurse, I forgot to check out my new-look boob and was already dressed before it dawned on me. So when we arrived home, I could wait no longer.

I dropped my bag in the kitchen and hurried upstairs to the bathroom mirror. I pulled my T-shirt over my head, unhooked my bra and hesitated. HoN had followed me into the bathroom, and when I caught his eye in the mirror, he smiled encouragement. He had read enough to know this moment was very significant for a woman who had undergone a mastectomy of any size and, once again, he was ready to be my support.

As my bra dropped to the floor, my eyes were focused entirely on my left breast. I examined the stitch marks at the tip of my breast and could see what a neat job Sir Clive of Clusters had done. My eyes then travelled to my right breast and it became apparent how much of my left breast had been taken. My eyes slid between the two as I compared my altered shape, but then suddenly I leant closer to my reflection, and frowned.

'Where's my nipple gone?' I said, stunned by this discovery. 'I look...sort of...I don't know...weird.'

HoN put his hand on my shoulder as he met my gaze in the mirror. 'The doctor did warn you about that,' he said, watching my reaction closely. 'He said they would have to take the nipple and quite a bit of the breast.' He looked concerned. 'Don't you remember that conversation?'

I didn't. It must have been one of those times when I chose to shut down – to not hear what I was unable to deal with at the time.

I stared at my misshapen breast trying to associate it with me and my whole image. For the size of the lump, which was no bigger than your average pea, they had certainly taken quite a large portion of the breast. The end of the breast had been stitched in a circle and then the thread (or whatever they use) had been drawn in like a purse string, so it gave the end of the breast a somewhat puckered look.

'My God,' I screeched. 'It looks like a cat's arse!"

HoN and I exchanged glances in the mirror and suddenly my face broke into a smile. HoN grinned, and the next minute we were both bent double laughing at my new look.

'Doesn't really match Won Hung Lo on the right any more,' I

spluttered, tears of laughter running down my legs. But then the impact of losing half my breast hit me and, as the smile faded, I stared at my uneven pair.

I had longed for smaller boobs most of my life, and hated the nicknames given to me which referred to my more than adequate cup size. Sure, I did a pretty good job of hiding my hurt – people wouldn't have teased me had I not laughed along with them.

This whole 'big bazookas' thing was certainly hereditary, as my own mother had had breast reduction surgery when she turned fifty, and the change in her, both physically and emotionally, was quite marked. I had toyed with the idea over the years, but each time I thought about contacting a surgeon and discussing it, I always had the problem of having surgery, and therefore anaesthetic, when it was not medically necessary.

'Are you sure you're OK?' HoN asked, as he wrapped his arms around me, concern coating his words.

I met his eyes in the mirror for a few moments and then returned his smile. 'Yeah, I'm cool,' I said, and I was telling the truth. Because his eyes had told me all I needed to know. When you are made to feel beautiful, nothing else is important.

Friday 5 October

Today was a big one – my first chemotherapy treatment. I was surprisingly calm. I say 'surprisingly' because I'd been feeling apprehensive about the whole thing for a number of days, knowing that, by going ahead with this, I had just given the nod to allowing toxins to be introduced into my body. In the end, however, I didn't see there was a lot of choice – I had more life to live and more books to write. But as I lay in bed last night, my predominant thought was 'The sooner I start this, the sooner it's over and done with.'

I didn't have time to dwell on it this morning either, as friends and relatives kept me busy with messages of good luck, and they did wonders for my attitude. With so many people thinking of me, how could I let them down? HoN insisted on driving me there and while I agreed to that, I was determined to cope with the treatment alone. I don't know why, but it was just something I needed to do by myself. But as I walked into the day care treatment room at the hospital, I suddenly felt like the new girl. I was transported back to my first year at college.

Our family had moved interstate through my father's new job and this meant starting school in Melbourne a few weeks into the second term, when friendships and cliques were already well established. That exercise found me transformed from a confident, always in charge, too much to say for herself girl, into a shy, incoherent nobody I failed to recognise as I stood at the front of the classroom with the headmaster performing an introduction and twenty-five sets of eyes assessing me.

Thankfully there were fewer people in the treatment room, but the eyes were still curious with questions. The one familiar face was Sophie, the clinical nurse we met in the oncologist's rooms, and her welcome was wonderfully warm.

It was an intimate atmosphere with only five recliner chairs for patients. That in itself was a shock, as I had expected a larger room, with rows and rows of people hooked up to drips, all at various stages of treatment. And why didn't they have a curtain around each chair for privacy?

I was suddenly grateful for the bag I was clutching in my left hand. It held a sudoku puzzle book, the current novel I was reading and a portable DVD player and disc of a favourite British comedy series. Oh yes – I was going to keep myself to myself. After all, the last thing I wanted to do was compare cancer stories with the other patients. One of the things I remembered the oncologist saying was 'Everyone's journey is different.' But as I sat concentrating on where the numbers from 1 to 9 fitted in the 81 boxes of my sudoku, I felt the woman in the next chair looking at me.

'Is this your first treatment?' she asked.

'Yes,' I said, giving a quick smile, before turning back to my puzzle. But then I felt her eyes still on me. I looked back at her, and the need for companionship was like a cry for help.

I put my puzzle book down and leant back in the chair. 'How about you – first treatment as well?' I asked.

She nodded, and leant closer. 'Are you frightened about losing your hair – or is it just me?'

'No, I don't think you're alone there. It is going to be weird seeing ourselves bald,' I replied, unconsciously bonding with this new friend. 'I think I'm more worried about losing my eyebrows and eyelashes. You can't fight that with wigs and scarves.'

She looked distressed, and I immediately felt contrite. She had obviously not thought through that next step in the hair loss scenario, and here I was literally hitting her in the face with the reality of our treatment.

'Actually, my cat's getting quite nervous lately,' I quickly said. 'I keep following her around collecting the fur she's shedding for summer. But I'm not totally convinced that silver tabby eyebrows are going to be a trendy fashion statement.' At least that comment brought a smile to my new friend's face.

'It may sound strange, but I'm kind of looking forward to losing my hair,' I added. The look she gave me indicated I might have been not just strange but completely insane!

'It's just that my husband suggested I prepare well before the hair loss happens,' I explained, 'so we did the wig and scarf thing a few weeks ago. And now I've bought so many scarves, there's probably none left in metropolitan Adelaide.'

She smiled, but then leant her head back and closed her eyes. She had had enough sharing.

Now I had opened myself up to the room and its occupants, a conversation between another patient and one of the nurses caught my attention.

'I had two lumps removed,' the patient said, 'and my surgeon told me that one was sent for research here in Australia, and the other was sent to Holland.'

What? This was something I hadn't even contemplated – that something happened after the 'coming out party'. Oh sure, I knew all the D'Lumps were taken away and analysed, but I didn't realise some of these lucky lumps won an overseas holiday. I wondered where Delores had ended up. It's not the sort of thing I had thought to ask my surgeon. But then again, did I really want to know? How would I feel if Delores had just been dumped? Maybe it was better her destination remained a mystery.

It seemed to be ladies club today as all five recliners were occupied by women. One of them had her husband sitting at her side, and her tetchiness cut through the air.

'Ask her if she can check my drip – it doesn't feel right,' she said to her husband, pointing at the other clinical nurse.

The nurse overheard her, and smiled at the husband. 'I'll be there in a moment.'

The husband asked his wife if she needed anything from the kiosk.

'I told you five minutes ago that I wasn't hungry – and no, I don't want anything to drink either,' she snapped.

My heart went out to this loyal man. He was obviously

trying to help her in any way he could and she didn't seem to appreciate it at all. But suddenly she leant her head back and closed her eyes. A few minutes later, her breathing was heavy and it was obvious she had fallen asleep. Her husband noticed me looking her way.

'Poor darling, this is her second to last treatment,' he whispered. 'She's been so good up until now, but I think it's just starting to get to her. Plus she's not sleeping well.'

It was like being doused with a bucket of cold water as I realised my journey had only just begun. I was still embracing this new adventure with a positive outlook. But would this be me in a few months time?

And then Sophie walked over to my chair dressed in goggles and protective smock, and it was like a lightning bolt – we were dealing with some pretty dangerous substances. Another reality check!

Sophie smiled and pointed to the empty drip bag. 'That's one lot down, Claire,' she said, hooking a new bag onto the stand. 'Now for the colourful stuff!'

I had been told that one of the drugs turns your urine pink. Must be where they get the idea of pink for breast cancer! I was eager to see if this was true, and this bag didn't take as long to empty, so I couldn't wait to head off to the toilet to check it out.

But when I returned to the treatment room, I stood at the door and addressed the other patients. 'OK, confess, you lot. Who can honestly say they had pink wee? Mine's more a tangerine, which really annoys me, as it doesn't go with anything in my wardrobe!'

We laughed at our common bond.

Oh yes, I was going to keep myself to myself. And wasn't I doing a good job?

Monday 15 October

I'm so tired. It seems to overwhelm me by the afternoon and this is only after one treatment. I was told that my tiredness would increase with each chemotherapy date, so I can only assume that by the end of my treatment, I'll be fully comatose! I'm having a few dizzy spells but this could be attributable to broken sleep. As I lie in bed, I can hear my heart beating hard and the throb seems to echo in my head. I wonder if this is too much stress on my heart.

I had some really strange dreams last week, but the one that stays in my head was possibly the weirdest. I dreamt I was lying on the bed when a young boy came through the ceiling carrying a list of tide times for the local reef around his neck. And just to add to the weird factor, my grandmother was squatting on the blanket box trying to get away from a Maltese terrier. What in hell's teeth do they put in those drugs?

I had a really frightening incident happen to me this morning. I'd just stepped into the shower and was reaching for the soap, when my vision blurred. I blinked several times but it wouldn't clear, so I steadied myself against the shower screen glass and tried not to panic. I was sure that if I stood perfectly still and concentrated on a single item in the bathroom – I chose the toilet as I felt my life was heading there – my sight would return. But that wasn't going to happen. Not while I still had my fogged-up glasses on my nose!

And when the air conditioning repairman arrived this morning with a new grill, and I could only tell him that it will be nice to have 'the place fixed where the breeze comes through the roof', I knew that 'chemo vagueness' was not just a myth but had hit this little black duck with a vengeance. But today, it was important to overcome the tiredness as I had an important date.

In amongst the forest of information leaflets I had been given over the past weeks was a brochure advertising a 'Looking Good Feeling Better' workshop. These were organised to teach patients how to cope with a changing image as their hair fell out, along with their eyebrows, eyelashes and self-esteem. You are encouraged to bring a friend, and although the friend I wanted to share this experience with works full time, she didn't hesitate to take the morning off.

The minute we walked into the room, however, I wanted to turn round and run out. Most of the other participants had already arrived, and as I glanced at the other workshop participants, I had one thought only. 'I don't belong here – some of these people look really sick.'

I felt such a fraud. No wonder people kept telling me I looked well – compared to this lot I was bursting with good health! The patients sat at an oblong table in front of their name tags and the friends were asked to take a seat around the perimeter of the room. Why allow us to bring a friend and then separate us? No, this didn't augur well.

Just as I was weighing up the benefits of saying to my friend, 'Let's get out of here, have a coffee and you can go to work so you don't waste half a day's leave,' the woman running the workshop introduced herself. She was pleased to see us here and hoped we would benefit from what we learnt, but I wasn't having a bar of it.

'I don't belong, I don't belong' was like a mantra chanting in my brain. Several women had removed their hats and scarves and were displaying various stages of hair loss, and I hoped I wasn't staring in horror. Yes, horror. Of course I'd seen chemotherapy patients before, but this time I was being faced with my immediate future.

'Ladies, you'll notice in front of you a selection of cosmetics that have generously been donated by various companies. These are yours to use now, then you can take them home with you. If the colours are not right, it's not our fault. It only means you've given us the wrong information on the forms you were asked to send us.'

'Why would anyone give the wrong information – that doesn't even make sense?' I thought. But when I looked up and Teacher was staring at me, I realised I had actually said it out loud. Bugger!

'I'm sure I don't know,' she said, her mouth resembling an animal's rear end, 'but people do,' she said, dismissing me with a look, before she concentrated on the good pupils of the class. 'And now, let's take our make-up off, and I'll show you how to put it on properly.'

OK, let's think about this. I'm in my late fifties and I've been wearing make-up in some form or another since I was fourteen. By my reckoning, that's a hell of a long time. Don't tell me I've been doing it wrong all that time! (I said 'DON'T tell me!)

'Oh well, I'm here now – I may as well get into the spirit of this thing,' I thought, as I wiped cleanser off with a tissue. The make-up supplied was from some of the top cosmetic companies and I was anxious to see how they worked. I smoothed on the foundation, dusted on the blusher, highlighted my eyebrows and was just debating which colour eye shadow to use, when a voice cut the air.

'Ladies, if you would now pick up your foundation and, using it sparingly, dab a very small amount on your forehead, across your cheeks, nose and chin.' She glanced at me. 'And please do not go ahead without me. We must all stay together in this.'

Yeah – right! Everyone knew by now who the class reprobate was because Maxine Factor was staring straight at me. I glanced at my friend and made a face and she was a picture of self-control – almost. Eventually we all had 'faces' on and it was time to address the wig and scarf situation. Another woman stepped to the front of the room and took over. When she asked for a volunteer, there was dead silence, and I was tempted to offer my head, but then I knew it would be better for one of the women who had already lost her hair to be the model.

'Would you like to see what a wig looks like on you?' the woman asked an elderly lady with only a few wisps of her own hair left.

All morning my eyes had kept straying to this particular woman, as she seemed to epitomise everything I dreaded about cancer. Her skin was grey and stretched tightly over her slight frame. Her eyes looked much too large for her face and the few wisps of hair remaining clung to her scalp in one last valiant effort. She nodded shyly, but as the wig was placed on her head, a few adjustments made and a mirror held up in front of her, the woman's face transformed.

'Oh – oh – I look so different – it's lovely – I feel different – nice.' She couldn't wipe the grin from her face.

And that's when I realised my mistake. As cancer changes the inside of your body, the changes are reflected on the outside as well. You look in the mirror and wonder where your old self has disappeared to. But I had come to this workshop too soon. I still had a full head of hair. I hadn't really accepted that I was going to lose mine, and here I was being forced to confront this fact.

Yes, the workshop is a great idea, but it must be the right time. This woman had chosen her right time – I hadn't.

Saturday 20 October

My hair is all I think about lately. I stand in the shower and reach for the shampoo, then hesitate. I have never been reluctant to wash my hair in the past. In fact, I would do it every day if I could be bothered with the drying and styling. But I have it in my head (no pun intended) that my hair is going to fall out faster if I wash it, and I'll be left with a pile of blonde bubbles on the tiled floor. Even now, I only have to run my fingers through my hair, and I'm left with rather hirsute palms.

My scalp has started to feel a little uncomfortable. You know the feeling you get when you've parted your hair on one side for years then decide to change your style – the hair follicles object to being guided in a new direction. Perhaps all the little individual hairs realise what is about to happen and are hanging on for grim death, even though they know the battle will eventually be lost.

When I was first diagnosed, one of the most difficult things for me to cope with was being totally out of control of the whole situation. This cancer had taken over my body and was dictating what I should do and how I should handle it. But here at least was a situation where I could take back part of that control. I decided I was not going to sit quietly back and watch the rest of my hair slowly part company with my scalp. I was desperate to avoid the 'tufty' look I had seen on several women at the Looking Good workshop, so the decision was made. It was going to be a case of 'hair today, gone tomorrow'. I would have my head shaved. I picked up the phone and dialled my hairdresser.

Jill had been through this exercise with several of her clients over the years and understood my need for privacy. It's all very well to decide you are going to shave all your hair off, but I didn't see it as a bonding experience with a dozen total strangers in a suburban salon.

'I'll come round Friday night after work. Is that OK?' she asked.

I had been diagnosed with cancer, had a second operation, was told about the compilation treatment and had my first chemotherapy session, all on a Friday. Suddenly this day had slipped from my favourites. Why not!

As we waited for the knock on the door, HoN could tell I was a bit nervous about the whole operation. There would be such a dramatic difference to my look and I had changed my mind at least a dozen times about the big shave-off over the past few days. But then I kept seeing visions of a head with a few pathetic wisps of hair sticking out at odd angles, and knew I was making the right decision.

'Let's have a drink while we're waiting,' HoN said, holding up a bottle of bubbly which had appeared like magic.

He was obviously more prepared for this event than me, and I quickly agreed. The first two glasses hardly touched the sides and by the time my 'scissor sister' arrived, I was feeling remarkably relaxed and ready for anything. But was she?

'Are you sure you're ready for this, lovey, because it will be a shock, you know?' she said, looking deeply into my eyes.

'Yep, lop the lops,' I slurred, grinning at my hysterical humour. 'No, hang on – I meant lop the locks.'

She looked at HoN. 'Are you ready for this?' she asked.

He nodded. 'Yep, I can't wait,' he said, handing me a third, or was it a fourth, glass of bubbles.

As the buzz of the razor ran across my scalp, I watched HoN's face for any negative reaction, but I needn't have worried.

As the final razor swoop was completed, his face broke into a broad smile. 'You look beautiful, babe – I knew you would.'

Still not sure whether he was giving me the reaction that was expected, or being totally honest, I frowned. 'You can say what you really think. It's CK – I can take it.'

But almost before I'd finished the sentence, he had grabbed the mirror and was handing it to me. 'See for yourself. You have a great-shaped head – no bumps or lumps.'

The first glance was a shock. You don't realise how much of your essence lies in not only your facial expressions, but the hair that surrounds that face. I felt completely vulnerable, open, naked, and couldn't stop staring at the person looking out of the mirror at me, although she was a tad blurry round the edges!

So this would be life till about May next year – the look I would carry right through the heat of summer. Would I feel confident swimming without a head cover? Should I buy a bathing cap? Shriek! Not one of those colourful ones with rubber flowers all over them. I'd look like a leftover from a 1950s Esther Williams spectacular. Maybe I could add a peg on my nose and pretend I was a member of the synchronised swimming team; I would have to practise my ability to dive in and surface two seconds later with a smile on my face, however. And then I remembered all those beautiful scarves and turbans waiting upstairs. It was going to be a busy weekend.

We finished off the champagne, and after taking an inordinately long time to arrange a scarf around my head, I went out in public as a 'baldie' for the first time.

The video shop was busy and as we wandered across to the new releases, I noticed several people's eyes stray to my head scarf and it suddenly became clear. Up to this point, my condition had only been shared with relatives and close friends. Now I might as well be wearing a banner declaring my cancer to the world!

HoN must have picked up on my self consciousness and put his arm around me. 'I really mean it, babe – being bold suits you.'

Although HoN was born in England, his parents came to Australia when he was only three years old, so he is an Aussie through and through. But there are a few words he uses which give away his British origins. And 'bald' is one of them. I decided I loved his pronunciation because, thanks to him, I felt beautiful in my 'boldness'.

Friday 26 October

Some of the side effects from the chemo cocktail are not too dramatic when you take them individually. The numbness in my toes, fingers and tongue is strange more than anything, and I seem to have left my tastebuds back in the treatment room. My gums get quite sore due to mouth ulcers but this only worries me when I eat. But put these together with the diarrhoea, dizziness, earache and breathlessness and, over the past weeks, I've felt like crap. All these symptoms did eventually abate, but that was only a few days ago. And today it's time for treatment number two!

The first chemotherapy session three weeks ago went quite smoothly so I was feeling relaxed as I headed to the hospital this morning. That was, until I realised my 'angel', the doe-eyed Sophie, was having a day off. The clinical nurse looking after me had the same friendly manner, but this morning every chair was occupied, and there were even several patients waiting, so she was run off her feet. But finally it was my turn in the Jason recliner.

Most of the drips are inserted in the top of the patient's hand and this has the same effect on me as someone dragging their nails down a blackboard. When I asked if they could use some other area for the drip it was pointed out that, as the veins are more prominent in the hands, it is easier to insert the drip. The veins in my hands have never been too attractive and I can remember my eldest son, when he was quite young, pointing to my hand, which was displaying a rather prominent purple vein, pulling a face and saying, 'Yuk, Mum, that's so gross!'

So I was very surprised to find that today the nurse seemed to be having problems locating an accommodating vein After she had inserted and removed the drip several times, I was more than ready to call it quits. And even when she finally inserted the drip and decided this was the place it could stay, I didn't share her confidence. It felt wrong, and the machine the drip was hooked up to agreed with me, as the alarm constantly beeped throughout the morning. (This alarm sounded if the fluid was not feeding in to the vein properly.)

'Make sure you sit perfectly still,' the nurse said, after checking the drip yet again. 'It seems to go off if you move your hand even slightly.'

That did it! I wasn't about to move even an eyelash. In fact, I was so still I wouldn't have been surprised to find birds flying in through the window, sitting on my head and crapping on my face! I was even too afraid to pick up my book and read just in case the movement of my eyes skimming the pages set off the beep. I just sat there willing my hand to stay still, until all the drugs had been administered and the drip was finally removed. I couldn't wait to get out of there and didn't even say goodbye to the other familiar faces who had their treatment on a Friday.

As soon as we arrived home, I lay down to rest, grateful it was all over for another three weeks. But about ten minutes later, reality hit. The birds may have missed me in the treatment room, but judging from the after effects of the previous treatment, it was almost guaranteed they would be dumping a load on me within about forty-eight hours.

Monday 12 November

What a weekend we've just had! Last night, I couldn't wipe the smile from my face. It's a great concept, A Day on the Green. You travel to a winery – this time it was Peter Lehmann's in the heart of the beautiful Barossa Valley less than an hour's drive north of Adelaide – sit around with good friends, good food and good drink, listening to live music. And this weekend, 'live' was the operative word. I say 'sit' around, but once the music started, and Jimmy Barnes uttered his first unmistakeable note, we were up on our feet unable to stay still.

When we realised the length and harshness of the treatment I would be going through, HoN suggested we pinpoint dates along the way to afford special treats – something to aim for and revel in the anticipation. So when Jimmy made a date in the valley, we decided to be there. And not just for the Day – we set aside the whole weekend.

We've known the couple who accompanied us for many years, and always have lots of laughs when we're together. Margie had booked into a highly recommended restaurant on the Friday night, and it lived up to the rave reviews. But Saturday was going to be a big day, so we said our goodnights relatively early. The next morning I dressed in a favourite outfit, tied a hot pink silk scarf round my head and was more than ready for our fun day when the tour bus pulled up out the front of the hotel.

As soon as we decided on this weekend, we decided to do the thing properly. And wasn't that the right decision! A beautiful sit-down meal was laid out in a special marquee, accompanied, of course, by just the right wines. And when you finished your meal, seats had been arranged outside on the lawn, with a great view of the stage. Although I have to admit, we did end up down the front near the stage, punching the air, dancing and generally reliving the gigs we went to as teenagers, well before the term 'mosh pit' had been invented.

Sunday was approached with a leisurely bent and started with a mid-morning swim in the hotel pool. And here was yet another challenge for me. I had previously made jokes about donning a rubber cap covered in flowers should I go swimming in my baldness, but now it was time to face that issue. I had been very careful to cover my head with matching turbans and scarves, and only HoN had seen me in all my 'nakedness'.

'I don't care,' I thought. 'I'm here to enjoy myself.' I put on my bathers, grabbed a towel, held my pin-head high and walked to the pool.

'You look great,' Margie said. 'No, really, you do, Claire.'

And that's why we have good friends. There were a few other hotel guests using the pool, and after an initial glance, they went back to enjoying their swim.

I love the water and only consider a holiday successful if it's around coastline or at least I have access to a pool. But this particular exercise took me back to the day I had my head shaved, donned a scarf for the first time and went out to the video store. Then, I was announcing to the world I had cancer, but this time I felt I was exposing more of me than I ever wanted people to see, and I felt so vulnerable. I purposely stayed in the pool for a leisurely swim, but my heart only resumed its normal beat when I got back to our room.

But all good things seem to have a price. I've woken up this morning really exhausted. Oh well, it won't hurt to have a quiet twenty-four hours resting as I've got a busy week cramming things in before I'm laid low with the next chemo treatment which is due Friday.

Friday 16 November

I've been an emotional wreck this week – 'coming over all unnecessary' as Mum used to say – with tears ready to spill at the drop of a hat. And Wednesday was the worst day.

When I tell people I volunteer at the RSPCA once a week, their first comment is 'I couldn't do that – those poor animals would break my heart.' I used to feel like that. But you can turn away from what's going on, because it is too devastating to see any animal in pain or frightened, or you can accept that, unfortunately, there will always be a need for a society such as this, and you can do your bit. Every day the rescue officers have to confront some horrendous cases and yet they keep going because they know the good they are doing.

Initially, when I started my volunteering, I would go to the animal shelter down at Lonsdale and walk the prosecution dogs. These are dogs which have been mistreated and need their confidence in the human race restored. This also gives them an opportunity for some exercise outside their cages.

But the last few years I have moved into the administration side of things and I now help at the city office. They do have an Animal House in the city, and welcome volunteers having contact with the animals brought in. All these darlings need as much TLC as you can give them but your contact is by choice not circumstance.

I can never resist having a chat with some of the animals brought in each day, but I have my own way of handling the heartache you feel. I tell myself (and the animals as well) that from this moment on they are safe, surrounded by people who will love and feed them, and may even be lucky enough to find a new home. But this week, when I stood in front of a cage which housed a mother cat and her four ginger kittens, I suddenly started sobbing.

The kittens were secure, curled against their mother's warm stomach. But the look in the mother cat's eyes was one of fear. She appeared terrified, probably wondering what would happen to her and her babies next. I wanted so desperately to reassure her that not only her babies were safe, but she was too.

As we drove to the hospital this morning for my third chemotherapy treatment, I remembered this cat's face and could almost relate to how she felt. But my terror came from knowing exactly what to expect and I was close to begging HoN to turn the car around and head back home. I wanted to scream, 'I can't do this any more.' I was frightened of everything – the injections, the toxins, the days of sickness ahead. I now hated Fridays. No longer were they the prelude to a relaxing weekend and time spent with family and friends. It was 'toxic tequila' day and frankly, I didn't know how much longer I could do this.

The thought of the discomfort as the nursing staff tried to locate a vein to accommodate the drip had been playing on my mind for several days, so the nervousness was at its peak by the time I walked into the treatment room.

But I needn't have worried. When I mentioned my reluctance to the nurse, she understood immediately.

'Would you like us to get one of the doctors to insert the drip?' she asked.

The relief on my face must have been enough response as, ten minutes later, the doctor located a vein and inserted the cannula. Not wishing to join in the patients' conversation this time, I opened my novel and started reading. But five minutes later, I wondered if the drip had been inserted correctly, as I seemed to be leaking fluid from my eyes.

'Oh, no,' I thought, 'please don't let me break down in front of the others. How humiliating would that be?' I subtly wiped the tears but the woman sitting opposite had already noticed.

'Don't worry, dear,' she said, giving me a gentle smile, 'it's usually me having a cry. I'm so emotional and it's good to know I'm not alone.'

I smiled my thanks and did feel a little better. But with her comment, I suddenly realised that we were all trying so hard to be positive. And that's bloody hard to maintain all the time!

Someone I came across recently who had been through breast cancer several years earlier told me she was fed up with people telling her to be positive. I thought it harsh at the time, but it seemed to be a standard phrase people use, and I'm sure I've been guilty of it in the past. The doctor, nurses and support staff had warned me there would be times during treatment when I felt like crying, that this was perfectly normal. While I nodded agreement at the time, I had never really accepted this.

'That's how others might handle it,' I thought, 'but I'm going to be strong and not let the bastard get me down.' But the bastard had!

And there was an added factor which was affecting my mood. This morning I received a phone call from my gynaecologist. She was concerned about a uterine polyp which had been bleeding and was keen for it to be removed.

'When would you like to have it done?' she asked.

I wanted to say, 'Hang on, can't we just concentrate on one end of me at a time?' but then realised each doctor has their priorities.

'Can I get back to you, Ann? I'll have to drag out my social calendar and see when I can fit in Pamela Polyp's Coming Out Party.'

At least there was one good thing. I would have another opportunity to wear my tiara at the theatre!

Sunday 25 November

I've never been this crook. I'm sure I'd remember it if I had! My third chemo treatment was nine days ago and even before I left the treatment room, I wasn't feeling too flash. By the evening, I had put in my apologies for a book launch I had promised to attend, and the week went downhill from there.

Every day the nausea and tiredness seem overwhelming and, initially, I was determined not to give in to it. This worked for the first few days. Each morning I made myself get out of bed and have a shower. I figured if I was dressed I wouldn't look as sick as I felt. But half an hour later I found myself crawling back into bed to hug either the bucket or the pillow. With all this lying in bed, there was plenty of time to think, and that can be a dangerous exercise, particularly when you have been advised not to look into the future.

'It's probably best to concentrate only on the treatment you are having at the moment, and we'll discuss the next phase when we're through this one,' my WWW (Wonderful Wicked Witch) had said.

Hang on – that's not how I run my life. I need to look ahead and plan, and from where I was sitting (or lying) I didn't like what the next few months held. I hated not achieving something each day. It didn't have to be a huge 'something', but at the end of the day just before I drift off to sleep, I like to be able to say, 'it was good I did that.' My one daily achievement this past week was being able to walk downstairs.

I find the nausea abates by late afternoon, and I can actually entertain the idea of having some food in my stomach. I had been warned by the nurses at the treatment centre that hunger was a side effect of one of the drugs, but I was amazed that one minute the thought of anything on a plate or bowl could make me vomit, and the next minute I was wondering what food was in the fridge.

But I don't want just anything. Oh no. I've actually become very selective. And it doesn't take an Einstein to work out that my food preferences are being controlled by the psychological rather than the physiological, because all I crave are the comfort foods of my childhood – the things Mum tempted me with on the rare occasions when I was ill as a child. Maybe this is a subconscious cry to be nurtured all over again, or maybe it is merely the sort of food bland enough to be ingested without being rejected two minutes later.

My daily diet at the moment comprises the following – Weetbix with warm milk (the cereal must not crunch) or Vegemite sandwiches (white bread only) or soft-boiled egg (with toast cut into soldiers – yes, it does taste different that way) or a particular favourite, extra mild cheese (the sort that tastes like soap!) and grated apple. And today I remembered my childhood penchant for junket. One of my happiest memories was staying with Gran and Grandpa while Mum and Dad went away and Gran made a different colour junket for every day of the week. I thought I had died and gone to heaven!

So there is light at the end of the daily tunnel – it's just that I have to run into a hell of a lot of trains to get there!

Friday 7 December

I reached the halfway mark today – four chemotherapy treatments down and four to go. Well, that's the A and C drugs. I'll still have to have the Herceptin administered intravenously, but apparently that one doesn't have the dreadful side effects.

One of the drugs made my sinuses feel blocked and my eyes sensitive, so I'm relieved to see the end of that! There's something else I'd be happy to see the end of and that is hot flushes, but this could be more to do with menopause and giving up hormone replacement therapy rather than the chemotherapy drugs. In my youth (and ignorance) I wondered why some women made such a big deal out of 'feeling a bit hot'. Little did I know that God was listening and decided to teach me a lesson!

From the moment menopause hit in my late forties, I suffered from flushes which left me throwing my clothes and my sanity out the window! Not only did I suffer hot flushes strong enough to power a small European country in the depth of winter, but the accompanying 'brain freeze' became serious enough to affect my work performance. It was after this that I regretted my previous insensitivity to other women, and rushed to the doctor. She immediately started me on HRT (helluva reliable tablet) and I had been worshipping at its altar every morning since. But with the suggested link between hormone replacement therapy and breast cancer by some areas of the medical profession, I was told to stop taking it as soon as the cancer was diagnosed.

And so the flushes were back with a vengeance! And it wasn't only me suffering. HoN often spends part of each night shivering and curled in the foetal position due to the bedcovers being hurled to the end of the bed in one of my roasting frenzies. When he can bear the cold no longer, he then sends out a search party for the quilt and bemoans this particular change of life – his, this time!

To cope with the daytime flushes (twenty-one at last count) I decided to take a leaf from my mother's book. I could remember her having a small mint-green battery-operated fan she would use at the first sign of a bead of perspiration. This caused me acute embarrassment when I was younger (the fanning, not the perspiring) as people stared when Mum revved up, but it's amazing how these inhibitions disappear as we turn into our mothers.

The twenty-first century version of the hand-held battery fan was a very different animal. It was sleek, black and compact and even gave you the option of programming messages which would then flash across the blades when the fan was turned on. I couldn't help wondering who decided that if you didn't get enough people staring at you when you whipped out your battery operated toy in public, you could grab their attention with a few well chosen words.

I wasn't going to bother with the message function, but the temptation for a bit of creativity got to me in the end. And what parent doesn't like to embarrass their children in public. Yes, too tempting to ignore!

'I'm a hottie' was the first message I programmed in. It was really stating the bleeding obvious because each morning, as I looked in the mirror, I knew, without a shadow of a doubt, the bald woman with lopsided boobs and no eyebrows would send the male population into a frenzy!

'A royal flush' was the next flashing message. This one was suggested by my youngest. Not, I hasten to add, because he thought I carried myself with a regal bearing. He just happens to be heavily into online poker at the moment.

'My fan club' was the final message. No one has asked to join at this stage, but if they're interested, membership is free. Just quietly, I'll pay you!

And I think I'd better stock up on batteries as well.

My aunt saw me fanning myself the other day and frowned. 'You poor darling! I think you'll find this runs in the family, dear. I still have flushes.' And she's ninety-four!

Tuesday 18 December

I've been awake for what seems like hours. Not sure how long it's really been as I've resisted turning my head and looking at the bedside clock. But the total absence of any sound at all tells me it's not even close to dawn. One thing's for sure – getting back to sleep is going to be almost impossible, as my mind has started ticking over. And it's always at this time that my thoughts head off on a sombre and depressing track and my positive attitude is nowhere to be found.

What if all this treatment doesn't work? What if I'm going through all this for nothing and the cancer comes back somewhere else? Maybe I should be making a list of things to do before I run out of time? Sure, I've been given all the positive statistics, but frankly, at this time of the morning, statistics mean Jack Shit!

But then I start thinking about my life and know I should be more grateful. What about the children and young adults who are diagnosed with cancer and the prognosis is poor? They will never have a chance to see their children grow up and go out into the world. Life has been good to me in a lot of ways, and I should be more grateful. But when you realise you might be facing your own mortality, you have a desperate need to grab hold of life by the fingernails and scream, 'I want more!'

Since diagnosis, I feel as if I'm living in the centre of an enormous bubble. This is a protective shell I've built, a small area which I can control. Providing I don't think about my condition too much (which means staying right in the centre of the bubble and just getting through the treatment) I'm fine. But then there are the times when I can't find the energy to centre, and I knock against the sides of the bubble. This ruptures the delicate membrane of my world, and allows reality to seep inside.

I had one of those moments this week. Everything was fine; I watched some television (from the centre of my bubble), and had even laughed till I nearly wet myself over a new program. But then, without warning, I was a blubbering mess. Depressive thoughts about my condition seemed to overwhelm me and I was crashing against the bubble's walls on all sides. It suddenly hit me. I didn't want to continue with the chemo treatment any more – I was sick of it – but at the same time I knew if I didn't continue, the chances of the cancer recurring were much higher.

It's halfway through my treatment, and I seem to be knocking against the bubble's sides more and more lately. Silly, isn't it? I was diagnosed with cancer nearly four months ago, and I feel as if it's only just impacting on me now. And one of the side effects of this impact is a lack of patience, which, heaven help me, I am directing towards HoN.

I remember my first chemo treatment when I sat listening to the wife who seemed to be berating her husband for everything when he was only trying to be kind and understanding. And here I was turning into her! Suddenly I understood how she was feeling, because I'm also scared, and we tend to take out our fears on the person we love most.

I turn my head on the pillow and watch HoN sleeping. I want to wake him up and apologise, but if it was a choice of sleeping till a respectable hour of the morning or giving his wife a chance to clear her conscience, I know which one he would choose.

Several people in the medical profession said the same thing to me, in different ways, and it really boiled down to one thing. Everyone's journey is different, so don't listen to other cancer patients. There is an enormous amount of sense in this statement, particularly when it comes to drug treatments and what is specifically recommended for you. But you will be told of other people and how they've coped, and it can't help but affect you.

I heard news the other day of a distant relation who was recently diagnosed with breast cancer. She is now on her third series of chemotherapy 'because the first two didn't work', and her prognosis is poor. How does someone cope with that?

But the celebrities who are diagnosed with breast cancer always seem to cope so well with this curve ball they're thrown. I think I need to know that in the privacy of their own homes that Kylie and Olivia and Jane sometimes threw themselves on their beds and sobbed uncontrollably. And maybe they also snapped at loved ones who tried to help them.

The physical journey is difficult but the emotional can be twice as hard. And wasn't this exactly what my surgeon told me in the early days of my diagnosis?

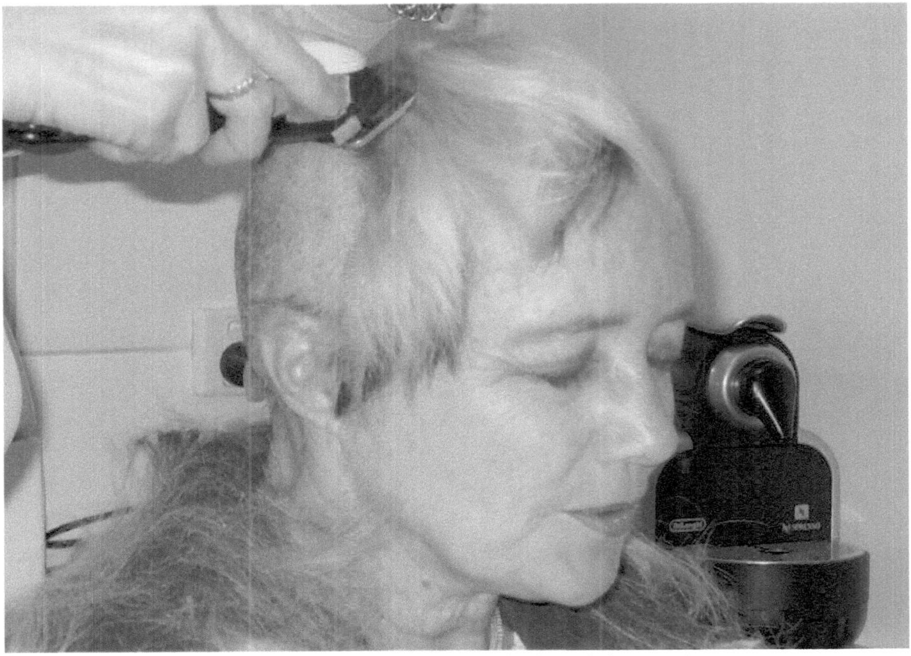

Hair today, gone tomorrow (through a haze of champagne)

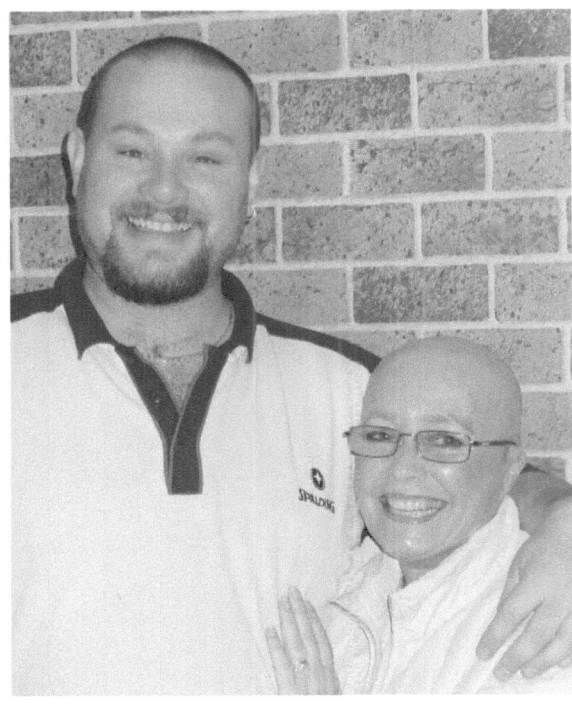

Like mother, like son (now all I need is a tatt)

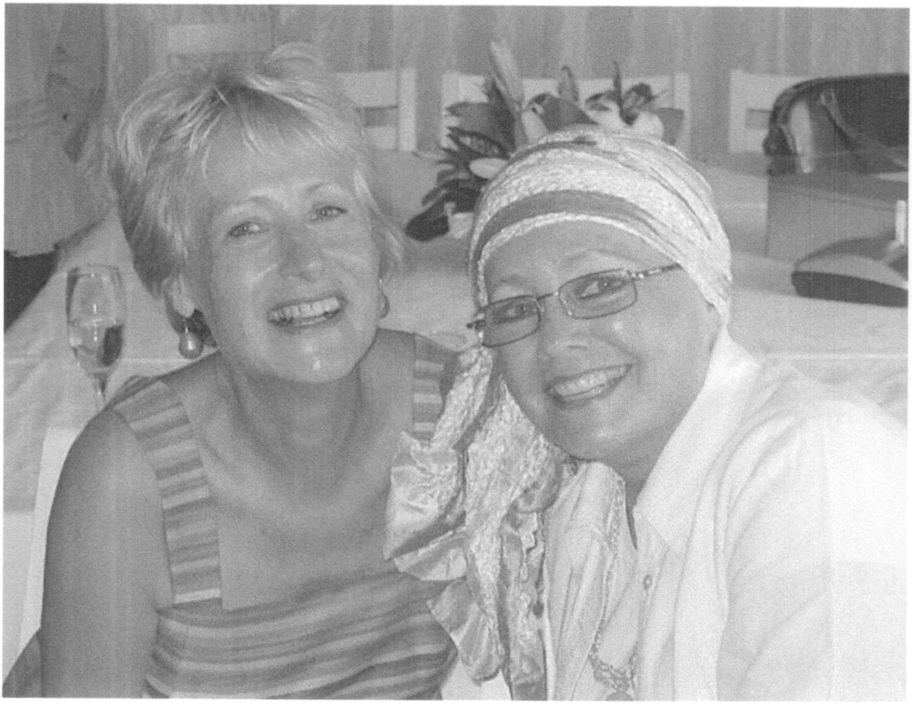

With dear friend Lyn Chaffey at her daughter's wedding (a respite from chemo)

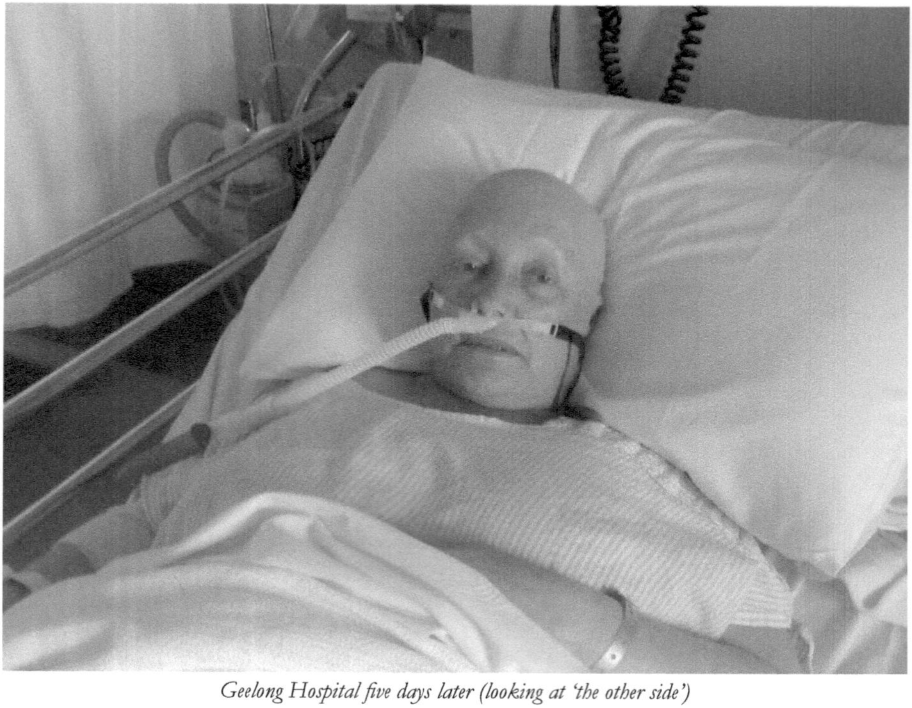

Geelong Hospital five days later (looking at 'the other side')

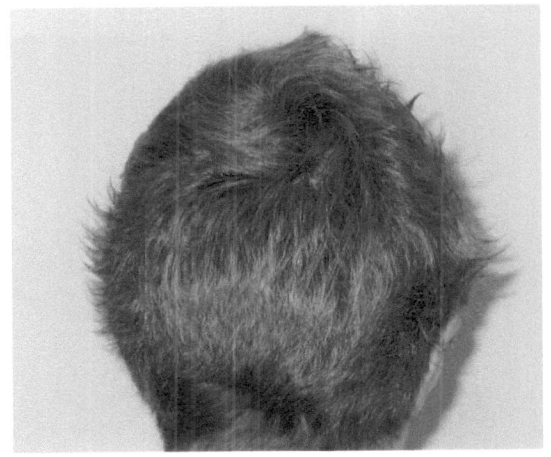

At last some hair again (but where's the 'natural' blonde?)

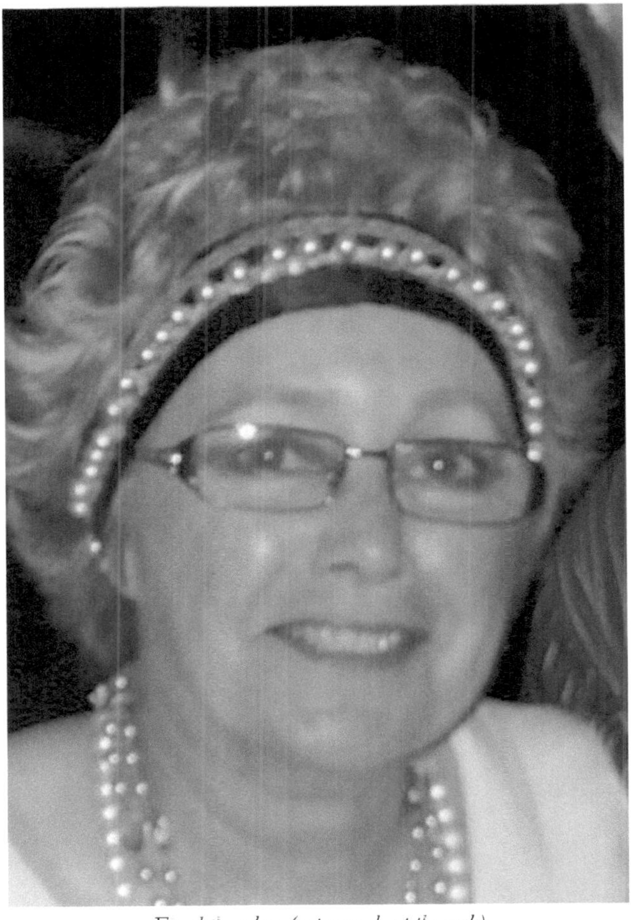

Fixed the colour (not sure about the curls)

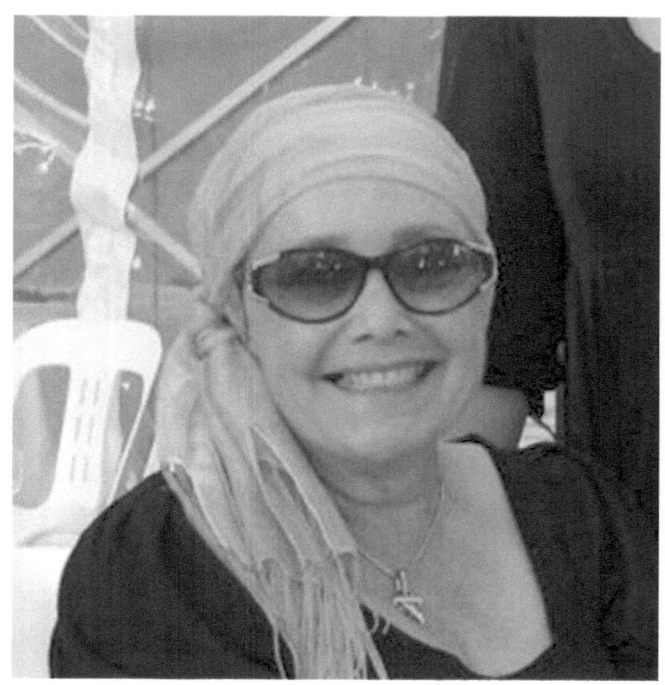

Day on The Green, Barossa Valley (Rockin' with Barnesy)

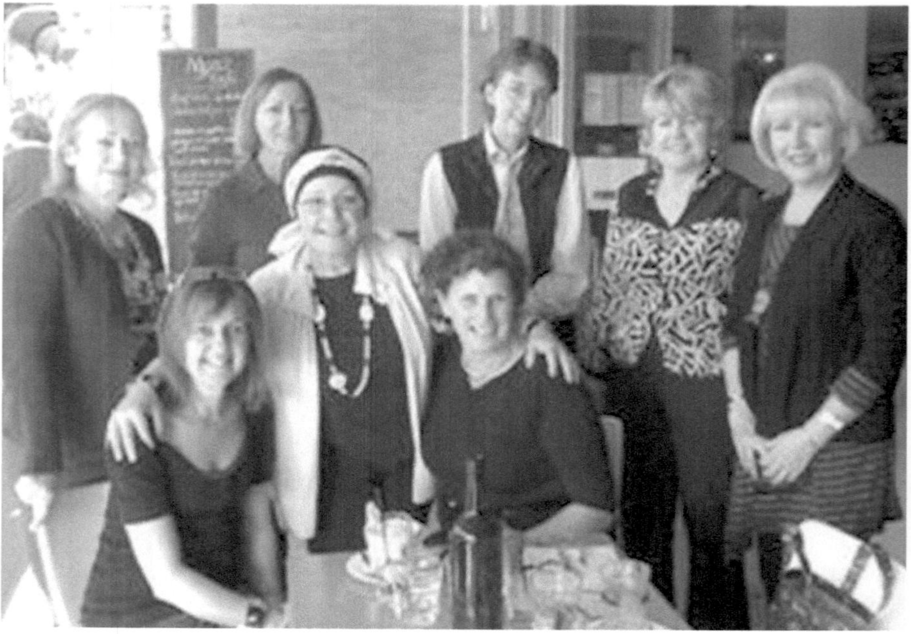

I get by with a lotta help from my friends

Thursday 10 January

I went to hospital again today, but this time I couldn't wait to get there, because I hoped the procedure I was booked in for was going to make my chemotherapy treatments less stressful. Each Friday I cringe as the nurses, and often the doctors, probe around my hand or forearm as they play the rather painful game I call HIV (hunt in vein) to locate a place to insert the drip.

But from now on, this particular problem should be solved, as I am now the proud owner of a port infusion which has been implanted in my chest. This port is connected by a slim catheter tube to a vein which goes directly into my heart. The port is an entry point for the drip which the nurse can use for administering the chemotherapy drugs.

But I was somewhat confused and more than a bit amused when I was told the doctor who had been recommended to do this procedure was a colorectal surgeon.

'Hang on,' I said to the nurse, 'aren't we looking at the wrong end?'

'No,' she said, smiling, 'he actually calls himself the ports and arseholes doc!'

It was only minor surgery, and after sitting in a waiting area with the other day trippers for about an hour, I found myself lying on a gurney in the corridor outside theatre.

A man in scrubs burst through a side door, and smiled down at me. 'Are you my next little cherub?' he asked, and I couldn't help noticing the devil in his eyes.

'Only if you're the ports and arseholes man,' I replied.

He grinned. 'That's me.'

'Actually, I think I qualify for both areas, doc,' I said, as he walked next to the orderly pushing my gurney towards the theatre. 'You may be putting a port in my chest, but this happens to be close to my left boob, and that resembles the arse end of a cat, so you'll feel right at home!'

He laughed. 'I can see we're going to get along famously.'

Although it only required a light anaesthetic, I still felt nauseous and dizzy when I woke up in recovery. And when I finally arrived home, the rest of the day and night was a blur of painkillers and ice packs. But I didn't really care. I had my port in the chemo storm and from here on, life was smooth sailing.

Thursday 17 January

I'm sharing my house with a complete stranger! Maybe not the entire house, because she only seems to confront me in the bathroom. Her mirrored image is unfamiliar, and it doesn't matter how many times I see it, I still can't accept the fact that this stranger is, in fact, me. I've heard the word 'featureless', and it's generally used to refer to something pretty boring. And how much are we defined by features like the hair on our heads?

When I first had my head shaved, there was a small amount of fuzz left behind – close to a guy's number one haircut. But now, even the last of the hair stubble has fallen off and I'm left with a 'chrome dome'. When I step from the shower and towel dry my head, if I stand in the right light, it has a real shine.

And that's only the start of it! I never realised how significant those small pieces of hair called eyebrows and eyelashes were – until I didn't have them! My face is a blank canvas which, in an artistic sense, is a chance for a new beginning.

But I don't want my slate wiped clean. While my face has the usual flaws, I've kind of got used to them and learnt how to live with them. Well, learnt how to disguise them with make-up is perhaps closer to the truth. And my eyebrows, in particular, have had their own history.

I can remember Mum washing my face when I was very young and running her fingers across each eyebrow. 'You're so lucky, darling, to have nice-shaped brows. You won't have to do a thing with them when you get older.'

This totally confused me at the time. I thought the only thing people did with their eyebrows was raise them. If I didn't have to do that, was life going to be easier?

So for the first eleven years of my life, I paid little attention to them. But then there was that Saturday afternoon when Mum caught me holding a pair of tweezers and gazing into the bathroom mirror.

'And what do you think you're doing, young lady?' she asked. 'You're not thinking about interfering with nature, are you?'

I hadn't thought of it in those terms, but yes, that's exactly what I was about to do.

She glanced at the tweezers, which had used up three week's pocket money. 'If you ever use those things, I shall have no hesitation in shaving all your hair off!'

Mum did have a love of the dramatic phrase, and in case that wasn't enough, the next day she presented me with something resembling a pixie's toilet brush.

'This is all I ever want to see you use on your brows,' she announced, before spitting on the bristles and trailing them across my hirsute forehead.

The thought of waking one morning to find myself bald scared me enough to give up the tweezer idea, but after her demonstration, the miniature toilet brush hit the rubbish bin. What is it with mothers and spit?

I'd like to tell you that eventually I grew up and told Mum I was going to make my own decisions regarding my body, but that would be a lie. I had to admit I'd lived with eyebrows au naturel for so long, I just couldn't be bothered doing anything about them any more.

It was pure coincidence, however, that I did start to think about getting my eyebrows waxed when Mum was no longer with us. I visited a local beautician to see what she could do with these two untrained friends of mine, and when I saw the result, I was ecstatic, but also slightly peeved. I had wasted all those years when I could have been looking this gorgeous from the age of eleven! But isn't timing everything? This only happened about a year before I was diagnosed with cancer and then I lost the lot. Mum had a long arm, but I didn't realise it stretched from heaven!

When I heard I would be losing my hair through the

particular chemotherapy drugs prescribed, I don't think I fully accepted it. Sure, I made a joke abut collecting the cat's fur for artificial brows, but the reality is a whole different ball game. When I stood in front of the mirror with a subtle shade of eyebrow pencil and tried to decide where to draw the line (my eyebrows, not my collecting of cat fur) it really hit home how important these features were in defining us as individuals.

And it was all very well to get the lines right first thing in the morning. But then, as the day progressed, I would forget about my drawn-on definition, and scratch or wipe my forehead and be left with one enquiring brown line, bereft of its matching twin – a fact I would only discover as I took my make-up off at night.

My eyelashes have been falling out for a few weeks now, and my eyes feel continually gritty. When I thought of lashes in the past, it was only ever how to curl or lengthen them and which mascara would give that come hither look. Now I was being reminded of their practical value and the real reason we had been given them in the prehistoric pre-cosmetic days.

And it's not only the face which acts as a constant reminder. When I stand in front of the mirror, my eyes travel to the area between my neck and my chest and are drawn to the yellow bruising and incision covering the slight lump at the top of my breast where the port infuser sits. The bruising will soon fade and eventually the port will no longer be required and can be removed, but I will always have the scar of the incision to remind me.

And then, of course there is the odd couple – the boobs that are no longer identical twins. One sister, although slightly shorter for her age, sits high and proud, but the other sister directs her gaze closer and closer to the floor. But I'm sort of used to them by now.

The rest of the body doesn't escape scrutiny either, but now I start to see the definite advantages to hair loss. It's such a drag getting rid of the foliage on legs, underarms and the little Tassie devil and, no matter which form of depilation you choose, it always seems to grow back too quickly. So take note, ladies – if you can possibly organise it, have your chemotherapy treatments during summer and you won't be leaving half your income at the local beauty salon!

It amazes and also frightens me, how something as small as Delores inside my body can have such a devastating effect and transform me on the outside as well. It's sort of like a double whammy – when your whole world has turned upside down, it seems the worst possible time for you to lose something as important as your own image.

Thursday 24 January

After the detailed analysis I went through about losing my 'look' last week, I decided it was time to think about other things. But that wasn't as easy as it sounded! I am still coming across people who are more acquaintances than friends so have yet to catch up with the news of my diagnosis. Like the other day.

I was heading home from work when I remembered I needed to buy a card for a friend's birthday. Stopping at the next chemist shop I came across, I darted inside and was standing at the card carousel, when a voice stopped me in my tracks.

'Claire, how lovely to see you after all this time. How have you been?'

I turned and recognised the woman who had worked at my local pharmacy for many years, and always had a smile to share.

'Cynthia – hello – so this is where you went!'

She nodded, then her eyes slowly focused on my head scarf. 'Bloody hell,' she said, frowning, 'don't tell me you've got cancer.'

I had received all sorts of reactions when people heard the news, but none had broached the subject as frankly as this. Some people really don't know what to say and my heart goes out to them as they dig around for an appropriate response. But in an odd way, Cynthia's openness was rather refreshing.

'Yes, I'm in the middle of chemo,' I said.

We discussed the treatment for a few minutes, and then she touched my arm and smiled.

'Well, you certainly don't look sick – just the opposite, really – you're quite plump and dewy!'

My face must have registered shock at such a description, and I thought I heard a loud thud as my jaw hit the floor.

Cynthia must have heard it too because she frowned and

waved her hand. 'No, no…oh God…I meant…er…that's really good,' she quickly added. 'You look soooo healthy.'

I smiled to relieve her anxiety, but I was still trying to grapple with the two adjectives I hoped would never be used in regard to my appearance – 'plump' and 'dewy'.

This wasn't the first time someone had commented how well I looked since commencing treatment. Everyone seemed amazed, including me, that you could actually look healthy when the chemotherapy drugs had to eat away at every part of you just so the cancer in your system was destroyed.

But when she said 'plump and dewy', all I heard was 'fat and sweaty'. This cocktail of drugs I was taking contained steroids, and I had been warned about bloating and fluid retention. And to add to this, between bouts of nausea, I was on a 'see food' diet!

In the days BC (before cancer), I had started a fitness regime. Yes, sounds impressive, doesn't it? In reality, this meant a twenty-minute beach walk each weekday and at least one longer walk during the weekend. Over the next few months, I could feel it doing me good. But then came the days AD (after diagnosis) when insanity invaded my world. And I never did get back to the walks.

And there's also that strange justification you bring into play when your world turns topsy. 'OK, I've just been told I have cancer and the treatment is on-going for quite some time. I deserve to have my special treats – no, bugger it, I can eat anything I want – there's more important things than being slim!'

That was the credo I lived by for the first few months, and before I knew it, the 'plump' was well established.

And the 'dewy'? Well, this came from the constant hot flushes brought on by having to give up the HRT (and we're not talking Holden Racing Team) and also some of the chemotherapy drugs. This meant waterfalls of sweat enveloping my whole body, particularly the face and neck.

Yes, I had to admit it. 'Plump and dewy' was probably accurate. I suppose she could have lied, but what was the alternative – thin and dehydrated? God, that sounded just as unattractive.

Yep, I guess the saying's right – we girls are never happy with our body image.

Monday 18 February

I stared at the computer screen, reading the email for the umpteenth time and feeling such a fraud.

> Hope today was still as upbeat as yesterday. You certainly don't mark time. I am plotting your trek over the mountain and you just keep marching no matter what challenges are laid before you. I am honestly full of admiration and your spirit is infectious xx Lizzie

Oh sure, I was fairly upbeat when I spoke to my wonderful friend over the border just before heading off to the hospital for treatment number twelve last Friday. These treatments are becoming so much a part of my life, and now that I have an infuser port, this makes treatments reasonably pain free and I can actually look forward to catching up with my fellow 'baldies'.

Saturday I was still feeling well and, yes, upbeat, probably because we had booked dinner and a show that evening. As I sat in Her Majesty's Theatre listening to the very funny Ross Noble and wiping the tears from my face, I had to agree that laughter was the best medicine. Then Sunday arrived and the chemicals kicked in and, along with my health, my mood plummeted.

Other friends had made similar comments about my attitude, using words such as 'optimistic' and 'inspirational', but the more effusive the praise, the guiltier I felt. On the surface it probably seemed as if I was taking this whole thing in my stride. I always find myself making a joke if a situation becomes too serious. I will never forget my parents arriving at my house one day both looking rather grim.

After glancing at each other several times, Mum took the

initiative. 'We've just been to the doctor and it's not good, dear. Dad's got cancer.'

I laughed – yes, laughed! Because I was so close to my father I couldn't stand the idea of anything being wrong with him. And certainly nothing as serious as this!

And I think another reason I have this reaction is that awful pregnant pause as you watch people's faces cloud over when you tell them bad news. You can almost see them grappling with a response – wondering what the right thing to say would be. It's only now that I fully understand there is no right or wrong thing to say. You instinctively know when people care, no matter what comes out of their mouths.

A common reaction when I first told friends of my diagnosis was nearly always the same. 'I am sooo sorry,' they would say, and I was often wrapped in a warm hug to show their support. After a few of these comments, I wondered at which level of serious information exchange we felt it appropriate to use the elongated 'o', as I myself had often done over the years.

I don't think we ever really stop and think about what our friends actually mean to us. If they do come into our thoughts, it's usually 'Must organise to catch up with so and so' or 'Wonder what they've been up to recently', but do we ever consider how eclectic our friendship base is and how these differences make each friendship special?

Their support was shown in many different ways. Some friends listen quietly as you explain the treatment you are having and others want to share information, their sentences beginning 'I knew a woman' or 'Did you see the article?' Then there are the others who are more adamant in their suggestions: 'Don't even consider' or 'Make sure you don't/do'. My earlier reaction, particularly to the latter suggestions, was a desire to say 'I don't want your advice', but now I view it differently. No matter how these friends react or what advice they want to give, the one thing they all have in common is their concern for me. And how could I be mad at that?

Emails and text messages are constant bursts of instant

support, but so are the cards carefully chosen, written, stamped and posted which look down on me from the fridge, whether it be through a kitten's gaze or a beautiful flower, both remind me people care.

One thing I am sure of, however, is that it's still easier on both of us if I'm optimistic when I talk to friends. But if I'm being totally honest, I really should admit one thing: being strong sucks!

Saturday 23 February

I started chemotherapy in October last year and the first four sessions were at three-weekly intervals and approximately four hours in length. It wasn't long before I really began to appreciate having that gap in treatment as it gave me valuable time to heal before the next lot of drugs hit my body. By the beginning of the third week, I was starting to get back some quality of life and for those next few days, I revelled in my good health. Just after Christmas, however, it was time to change drugs and Wonderful Wicked Witch advised these would be more effective if administered weekly.

The only thought I had when I heard this news was one of despair – now I'll feel like shit all the time! But if it was going to give me a better chance of getting rid of the cancer, I couldn't afford to ignore the doctor's advice. And I have to admit the last eight weeks, with chemo every Friday, hasn't been all bad.

The side effects usually don't kick in until the Sunday, so HoN would be there when I finished my treatment on the Friday and we would go out to lunch. I really looked forward to this treat. But inevitably, the side effects would eventually catch up and they were usually fairly overpowering and knocked me for a six. So yesterday, when I was due for treatment number nine, I didn't turn up. I ran away!

That's not quite as irresponsible as it sounds, although there have been many other Fridays I have been tempted to play hooky. In this case, however, it was an invitation to a wedding in Victoria that found me ringing the oncologist for a leave pass.

'As long as you make it up at the end of your treatment, I guess it wouldn't hurt,' my wicked witch said.

Apart from catching up with interstate friends I saw too

little of, this break was a chance for me to catch my breath (quite literally). Over the past month or so, I had been suffering constant breathless attacks which were brought on by even the slightest exertion. This is mentioned as one of the side effects of the drugs I am taking at the moment so I wasn't particularly alarmed and had learnt to pace myself (when I remembered!). But the breathless attacks did seem to be getting more frequent and certainly more severe.

The wedding is on Phillip Island, ninety minutes drive from the Melbourne CBD and because we've taken an extended weekend break, we opted for the scenic route along the Great Ocean Road. It's one of our favourite tourist drives and both HoN and I never get sick of the scenery.

Before we reached Philip Island, we caught up with friends who picked us up from the Sorrento ferry terminal and took us back to their beautiful beach house in Blairgowrie for lunch. All the excitement did take its toll, however, so yesterday was spent resting, preserving my energy for the big one.

And today is the wedding! The wedding invitation read 'Dress – Summery Picnic with Style' and I found just what I wanted the first day I went shopping. It was a taupe linen skirt and a linen top in pale pink and I even found the perfect matching sandals in taupe. But when I walked outside this morning, the sky looked ominous and the air was sharp with a distinct chill.

My heart went out to the bride – so much for her 'summery picnic' – but having known this particular bride since she was a little girl, I knew she wouldn't let inclement weather ruin her day. Luckily I had packed a long-sleeved jacket so I threw this over my linen top and reached for the sandals.

Several of my toenails had turned black a few weeks ago, so I had painted them with a fairly dark nail polish. But as I slid my feet into the sandals, I knocked the big toe on my right foot and nearly passed out with the pain. As I looked down, I realised my toe had become infected and there was constant discharge coming from under the nail. So much for my new sandals!

Why couldn't I just have this one day to completely forgot

about how screwed up my life has become? Sure, there was the fairly obvious reminder as I covered my bald head with a scarf, but it was the most beautiful scarf I had ever owned and had cost me nearly as much as the whole outfit!

And then there was the other constant in my life – the breathlessness. It took longer than usual to get ready and it seemed a lot more severe today. No, I didn't need any more reminders. But then I remembered – I was here to celebrate, not commiserate, so I whacked a Band-Aid on my toe, dropped a spare in my handbag, took a steadying breath and headed off.

Monday 25 February

I made it – I got through the wedding on Saturday! Unfortunately the bride and groom's hopes for a summery picnic wedding were dashed as the wind and rain relentlessly buffeted the large white marquee perched on the cliff top. It didn't seem to matter, as it turned out to be one of the most wonderful, casual and enjoyable weddings I have ever been a guest at. The bride's mother and I have been friends since we were in our early teens, and I've always had a place in my heart for her children, so this made it an extra special day.

One thing I wasn't prepared for, however, was the emotion shown by my friend when she first caught sight of me. Since I had told her of my diagnosis, she had sent her support across the kilometres in all sorts of ways. We spoke regularly on the phone and she was always checking on the progress of my treatment. But suddenly, there I was in person, a scarf covering my bald head, and the real impact of the situation must have only just hit home. Her eyes filled with tears as she wrapped me in her usual, warm hug, but after only a few moments, I forced myself to step back. I only wanted happy memories of her daughter's big day.

Perhaps I should have restricted myself just to the wedding. But the bride and groom put on a 'recovery barbecue' the next day as an extra opportunity for their guests to catch up with each other, and I was certainly not going to miss out on that. And then our other dear friends from Melbourne took today off work so we could have lunch together in Queenscliff. Yes, too many wonderful opportunities – how could I say no? And now I feel like shit!

The breathless periods are much more frequent and I feel

constantly exhausted. Haven't said anything to HoN, but I'm really scared and not sure this is normal. We have found a lovely little bed and breakfast in Apollo Bay for tonight, and I wish I could appreciate it more. But as soon as we stepped inside, I only had enough energy to make it to the couch and have been there ever since. I feel the need to take deeper and deeper breaths. Didn't even think to ask my wonderful wicked witch just how much breathlessness I should expect with the chemotherapy treatment. Perhaps I'll give her a call before we set off tomorrow. Now I know how a goldfish feels when it's robbed of its bowl of water!

Sunday 2 March

The goldfish finally ran out of water. We didn't make it back home – just the opposite actually – we ended up heading back in the direction we had already been.

As soon as I woke up on the Tuesday morning in Apollo Bay, I knew I was in trouble. I nudged HoN. 'Can't breathe,' I whispered, and the panic in my voice woke him fully.

He had been concerned enough about my diminishing health last night, so before going to bed had researched the local medical facilities and was prepared. 'Apparently there's a small hospital here – I'll ring and tell them we're on our way,' he said, throwing some clothes on and then helping me to dress.

It was less than five minutes drive from where we were staying and the night duty nurse, who was just about to finish her shift, greeted us at the door and summed up the situation.

'Let's get you on some oxygen,' she said, guiding me in to the small emergency area.

The relief was beyond description, and I took the first deep gulps of air I had breathed in days. Because of the early hour, we had to wait for a doctor to be summoned, but I didn't mind – I had air! I turned and smiled at HoN. His relief almost matched mine, and it was only then I saw how worried he'd been.

Eventually the nurse came back into the room, followed by a tall man with gentle eyes set in a face as black as the ace of spades.

After briefly catching up on my medical history and doing some tests, the doctor frowned. 'I'm sorry, but as you're an oncology patient, we're going to send you to Geelong Hospital. They have a much bigger facility there.'

'Hang on,' I thought. 'We're heading the wrong way. Surely I could stay here till I get my breath back, and then we could head home.' But somehow I didn't think this would be an option.

I glanced at HoN. 'Just as well you've packed the car already – we can head off straight away,' I said.

I was surprised to hear the doctor laugh. 'Not unless you've got oxygen in your car. No, you'll be going by ambulance. You need to be constantly monitored.'

I was ready to argue, but a lack of breath and a steely look from our medical friend left me with no alternative. I was about to travel the Great Ocean Road in the back of an ambulance. Bet that wasn't written up in any overseas tourist brochures.

The ambulance guys were fantastic – all four of them – as we had to change ambulances and crew at Lorne – but I did wish they would just stop talking. They kept asking how my breathing was and I was tempted to yell (although that would take too much breath), 'My breathing is fine AS LONG AS I DON'T HAVE TO TALK!'

But then we were pulling into the ambulance bay at Geelong Hospital and I was being wheeled into Emergency. I looked round for HoN but the area seemed full of hospital staff.

It turned into a very long day as different doctors were brought in to assess my condition. By late afternoon, the doctors and medical staff had run a myriad of tests. So many, in fact, that I was ready to lay bets I would pass one eventually, although that logic never applied with my education!

One of the first specialists I was introduced to was the oncologist, a rather gruff individual who didn't feel the necessity for manners (bedside or otherwise). He was thorough, however – a details man – and I would be extremely grateful for this over the ensuing days.

But in between gasps of air, I did manage to make one thing crystal clear to him. 'Please ring my oncologist in Adelaide and discuss treatment with her. I don't want anything done unless she agrees to it,' I muttered through the present oxygen mask, which was so large it covered my entire face.

One factor which was indisputable amongst the medical staff

was the build-up of fluid around my lungs, and this attracted the attention of three pulmonary specialists. 'Can't be much happening in the lung patient area today,' I thought, as Larry, Curly and Mo each took turns holding their stethoscopes on my chest and back, and gazing into the middle distance.

As the breathlessness could be attributable to several factors, it was necessary for the doctors to run a myriad of tests in those first twenty-four hours after I was brought in. I was too exhausted to care too much, but did feel a frisson of fear when I heard the words 'possible legionnaire's disease'. Didn't people get that when they were in hospital? And wasn't that what my friends' ex-neighbour died of a few years ago? Shriek!

Another thing the doctors were concerned about was the possibility of metastatic cancer, and if this was detected, it would mean my cancer had travelled from the breast and lymph nodes into other parts of the body. Perhaps I'll take the legionnaire's option!

The only test I actually smiled about was the one for PCP, a pneumonia you are susceptible to if your immune system is weakened. But wait a minute, wasn't that a recreation drug used at rave parties? The wedding on Saturday was great, but didn't quite fall into that category!

The final test was to ascertain whether I was experiencing a very rare and severe allergic reaction to one or more of the chemotherapy drugs. And eureka, it seems we had a winner. The culprit was a drug called Doxorubicin, the dastardly dox, and this brought on a condition called acute dilated cardiomyopathy. This is a disease of the heart muscle that causes the heart to become enlarged. The muscle becomes weak and unable to pump blood efficiently around the body and is called left-hand heart failure. It's ironic, really, because even before I started treatment, there were reservations in my mind about one of the other drugs called Herceptin, and what that would do to my heart. Hadn't I been concerned when I heard and felt my heart beating so loudly after one of the earlier chemotherapy treatments? Was that the first sign?

Although the prognosis was something which would affect me for the rest of my life, at that moment, it was a relief to give the condition a name. To me, there's nothing more frightening, in a medical sense, than not knowing what you're dealing with.

Now the doctors knew what they were treating, they were able to administer the appropriate medication over the next few days, and I started to gradually improve. But my attempts to remove the oxygen mask when Nurse Ratchett wasn't looking still found me gasping and grabbing for it a few seconds later. This particular nurse and I had crossed swords once before, when I begged her to take the mask off due to a panic attack and she refused. Just as well all the scalpels had been packed safely away!

Monday 3 March

Now the doctors knew what they were dealing with, they were able to work out a treatment regime, but indicated it would still be a lengthy stay in hospital.

My heart sank. This didn't really fit in with my plans at all. I had hoped that once the doctors knew what my condition was, they could give me some medication and we could head back along 'the yellow brick road'. But the stay in the intensive care unit did last until Thursday, so I had to acknowledge I wasn't feeling that flash.

HoN found a motel close by which he used as a home base and each day would visit bringing clean knickers and one-liners, both proving to save my sanity.

But one thing I was adamant about. 'I don't want you sitting by my bedside all day. Get out and have a look around Geelong, and then you can come here late afternoon and we'll have dinner together.'

While this was my way of expressing my deep love for this wonderfully supportive man, HoN demonstrated even more clearly the true depth of his love one day when the nurses were busy. He did bedpan duty!

On Thursday I was finally moved out of ICU (Insanely Claustrophobic Unit) and into a bright room with a lovely roomie. She was a young mother with a caring husband and two delightful children and this family proved to be just the diversion I needed. But this morning her doctor had been in and told her she was well enough to leave.

For perhaps the first time in my life, I was not instigating conversation with a complete stranger to find out what their story was – a habit I had inherited from my mother. I needed all my energy for the essential sentences like 'Can I take the mask off for just a while, please?' – this directed to the nursing staff – to 'When can I go home?' – a plea sent to any doctor game enough to stick his nose around the door. But my room-mate seemed to instinctively know when I needed some diversion, and would carry on a pretty much one-sided conversation.

We swapped email addresses, but I suspected she felt the same as me – once we left this artificial world and went back to our homes, our time together would become a blurred memory.

So I was feeling a bit lost. I lay there staring out the window focusing on the bit of ocean visible through the trees. The walls of the room started closing in on me and I wondered how long this nightmare was going to last. It's bad enough when you're very ill, but to be so far from home was way out of my comfort zone.

My teeth started aching, there was a buzzing noise in my head and I tried to take a deep breath as I felt the unmistakeable signs of a panic attack starting.

Just then, one of the nurses came into the room. 'We'd like to move you to a different room today,' she said. 'Things are a bit crowded so we're doing some shuffling.'

She smiled as though this was good news, but suddenly I desperately needed to hang on to something familiar. And the only move I was planning on making was the one through the front doors and out of here. I'd been creeping along my tether for a few days, but suddenly, I'd reached the end!

'No, I want to stay in this room,' I said, trying to sound firm, as my voice shook. 'Anyway, the doctor hasn't been around yet, and he may sign my release today.'

I was disappointed to see her frown as she left the room. 'Don't think I've convinced her,' I thought, 'but if I have to hang on to the doorknob, I'm not being moved.'

Ten minutes later, another nurse, who was fast becoming a friend, walked in and smiled at me. 'You're quite welcome to stay in this room, Claire, but we have to point out you'll be getting another room-mate, and the circumstances are a little unusual. This dear lady is extremely elderly and only has hours to live.

We're trying to find somewhere quiet for her and her family, but if it doesn't upset you, the family are happy for you to stay.'

I had the most unusual reaction to this bit of news – I had to suppress a smile. Please don't misunderstand – I'm not without sentiment or caring for situations such as these – just the reverse. My smile was at the thought of my friends hearing a room with me in it described as 'somewhere quiet'!

'No, that'll be fine, Jan. If they don't mind, I don't either.'

I had been with both my parents when their time was coming to an end, so I didn't fear the process of death. And I had also seen Mum and Dad after they had passed over, so there was no mystery there.

The curtain was pulled around the bed and the gurney was quietly moved into the room. Even if I hadn't been told she was elderly, the gentle strains of Vera Lynn singing 'The White Cliffs of Dover' coming from the tape deck next to her bed, would have given the game away.

I was transported back to the hospice where my father spent his last few weeks. Being a pianist all his life, the nursing staff had organised some classical piano tapes to be played to Dad when he fell into a coma. They say the last of the senses to go is your hearing, so why shouldn't you have the music which would make your heart soar?

Quite inappropriately, I suddenly had an insane desire to laugh out loud. I had just visualised HoN's reaction to my last musical request.

'Make sure they play AC/DC "It's a Long Way to the Top",' I'd say, even though I wasn't too confident this was where I'd be heading!

Several hours later, the elderly lady was still hanging on to life and I was hanging on to a wisp of hope. When the doctor did his rounds, I had made up my mind.

I turned on the biggest smile I could muster, and responded to his question. 'I feel sooo much better. If I promise to take it easy, could I be released from hospital today, do you think – please – pretty please?'

He stared at me for a few minutes. 'One proviso,' he said. 'I'd like you to stay here in Geelong for a few days before you attempt the trip home to Adelaide. You need to build up your strength. And when you do travel, only make it for a maximum of three hours per day. If you agree to that, I'll sign your release.'

Yes, anything – let me find you a pen. Watch out world, here I come!

'No problems,' I said, trying to contain my excitement. I couldn't wait to phone HoN.

It was all very well to put on a brave face for the doctor, but it was only when I got out of bed and started dressing that I realised how weak I'd become. And when we pulled up outside the motel room where HoN had extended his booking, the ten-second walk from the car to the room completely exhausted me and I was happy to fall on the bed.

When HoN went to the shops an hour later to pick up some supplies for the next few days, the emotions of the last few days finally spilled over. For the first time since I'd arrived at Geelong Hospital a week ago, I was beginning to realise recovery was going to take a long time. And for this recovery to be complete, I would need to find a component of my make up I was not terribly familiar with – patience.

Friday 7 March

We're home at last! In the end, the doctor's instruction to travel no more than three hours a day was easy to obey as my body just wasn't up to any more. Even though HoN had bought a dinky little blow-up pillow which wrapped around my neck so I could nod off comfortably while still sitting up – a position that helped the breathing – travelling still proved exhausting. And when we finally arrived at our destination each afternoon, the walk from the car to the motel room necessitated a rest on the bed for the next few hours.

This pace (or lack of) frustrated me no end. I've always moved from point A to point B at a pretty rapid rate, but this is one of the areas where HoN and I are poles apart. He is a stroller, a meanderer, and doesn't see the point (either A or B) in rushing anywhere. So here I was, clutching his arm and reduced to the walking speed of a sloth on annual leave, while my brain did an Eliza Doolittle and screamed, 'Move your bloomin' arse.'

As well as not feeling great, I found out I didn't look too great either. One day we had stopped for morning coffee at a café in a small town, when the conversation of four elderly women at a neighbouring table caught my attention.

'They say it really changes your whole outlook when you're diagnosed with cancer,' one woman said.

'Yes, it's probably that whole facing your own mortality thing people talk of,' another woman replied.

They then went on to discuss the subject further, and of course I was all ears.

After we had finished our coffees, HoN went over to the counter to pay, and I slowly shuffled to the door.

But just as I passed their table, I stopped and smiled. 'Sorry, ladies, I couldn't help overhearing your comments about cancer, and you're right – it does change your outlook. You relish every day,' I said.

One of the women glanced up at my head, and I felt embarrassed as I realised the small cotton scarf I had put on that morning was failing to cover my baldness.

'Are you having treatment?' she asked.

I nodded and she leant towards me. 'The reason I ask – and I hope you don't mind me saying this, dear – but there are workshops called Looking Good Feeling Better. They'll help you…' She paused, looking for the right words. '…feel…you know…sort of…better.'

There are times in your life when you experience two different reactions to the one incident. My first reaction when I heard this statement was one of horror! I must look pretty bad if a total stranger felt I was in need of some drastic help regarding my looks. But the second reaction found me desperately trying to suppress a laugh.

I suddenly remembered the great lengths (not to mention the great expense) I had gone through to enhance my new look, before even one hair had fallen to the floor – the copious amounts of scarves which had become an essential part of my wardrobe to hide my impending baldness. But when it came time to utilise these various pieces of coloured silk, there was one problem. When I had my head shaved by my hairdresser, she left a very light fuzz, even less than a number one, and this assisted in holding the silk scarf on to the scalp. But then after several more treatments, even that fuzz falls out, and you're left with a dome that looks as if it was polished with Mr Sheen. The scarf which previously was draped carefully over the head and tied in a bow under the right ear would only stay in place for a maximum of minutes. Any slight movement and the scarf would be sliding off and heading for the floor!

Having spent the equivalent of the gross domestic income of a small European country on headwear already, I needed a cheap solution to this problem. And that's how I discovered turbans, which gave the scarves something to hang on to. All it took was some T-shirt ribbing material in basic colours, a twist and twirl formula and the scarves stayed put.

And I soon found out that the SSS (Sliding Scarf Syndrome) was not only my particular problem. Each time I walked into the chemotherapy treatment room, it wasn't too long before I was asked about my head covering. And this wasn't always from my fellow baldies.

One daughter, sitting with her mother who was receiving her first chemotherapy treatment, therefore still maintaining her hair at this stage, looked across at me and smiled. 'I was just suggesting to Mum she ask how you do your turban. She's going to be losing her hair as well and hates the idea of a wig.'

And several times one or other of the clinical nurses would ask me to 'demonstrate' my turban to a new patient before I was hooked up to my treatment.

While I had no qualms about exposing my baldness (we were all in the same rocky boat), I soon realised that just watching someone 'fold, wrap and twist' may be much different to actually doing it at home by yourself. But then the problem was solved! I came up with a solution and, along with the demo, handed out 'how did she do that again?' sheets.

Da Chemo (W)Rap

Ya head it might be widdout da rug
And your brows and lashes missing from ya mug
But stick wit me I'ma showin' you how
To cope wid dis drama yo be learnin' right now

It's da chemo (w)rap and you can look good
When ya strut ya stuff in ya local hood
Follow the steps one to six an' you'll see
Just how easy dis nu look be

So go out now wit ya bran nu 'tude
Head held high you the main gal, dude
I promise you, girlfrien I ain't jokin'
Everyone ya meet will think ya smokin'

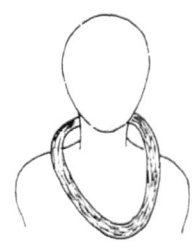 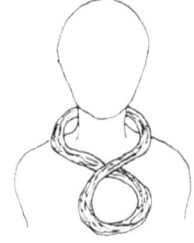 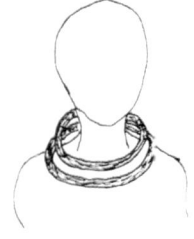

1. Slip loop of fabric over head and let it drape on chest.

2. Pick up loop and twist fabric into a figure eight.

3. Pull front loop back over head so you now have two loops round your neck.*

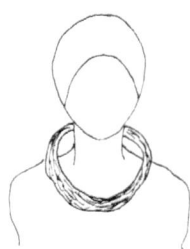 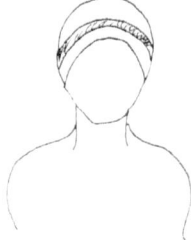 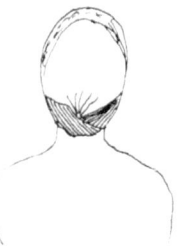

4. Lift loop closest to your neck over face and smooth over head to form skullcap. Fold rough edge back round face.

5. Keep remaining loop as a roll, lifting over face to form a band across top of head.*

6. Check back of turban in mirror to make sure ends tucked in.

* Fabric comes in different widths, so if you use larger ribbing material, you can make three loops.

And another thing which made this coffee-shop critic's words hard to swallow was the constant positive feedback I'd been receiving since starting treatment. So many people said to me 'You look sooooo well, no one would know you had cancer' and I was starting to believe it! But these comments were a while ago – well before 'the excreta hit the rotating device on the ceiling' and the doctors in Geelong had arrived at the 'heart' of the trouble. I suddenly realised an awkward silence had descended on the coffee clique, so I dragged up a weak smile.

'Yes, I did go to one – those workshop things – a while ago,' I said and, not being able to cope with the pregnant pause which followed, excused myself and headed for the door.

I could almost hear the conversation which followed my departure.

'Poor dear, she obviously didn't get much out of her particular workshop. Probably didn't pay close enough attention.' And she'd be right!

As we got back in the car, I shared the story with HoN and we both had a laugh. But when I pulled the sun visor down, flipped open the mirror and stared at my reflection, I suddenly saw what she was talking about. I had felt too tired and weak to even bother with the turbans and scarves since being admitted to hospital, and had made do with a small triangle of cotton fabric which barely covered my head. With my bald head and round, white pasty face, I was doing a fairly good impression of 'the only gay in the village' from Little Britain!

The final day we left ourselves a very short distance to travel and it seemed no time until we were making our way down the freeway through the Adelaide Hills. It had been a quiet trip as both of us were fairly exhausted by now, but as we reached the tollgate where you catch the first glimpse of the city of Adelaide, the dam of emotions I had controlled up to this point suddenly burst open.

HoN reached out for my hand.

'I didn't want to say it out loud before this moment,' I said, hiccupping with tears, 'but I didn't think I was ever going to see home again.'

Wednesday 12 March

I don't think I've ever been as scared as I was today.

Wait a minute, that's not entirely true. There was that incident when I was about nineteen and I'd just moved into a flat with my girlfriend. We shared a bedroom and although this did create friction (I was tidy, she wasn't) there was still comfort in knowing the other person was there.

This particular night something woke me up and when I glanced at the clock, I realised that, even though it was about three-thirty a.m., I was by myself – my housemate was still out partying. I was just about to turn over and try to get back to sleep when I froze, because there, behind the bedroom door, stood a dark figure. I opened my mouth to scream but no sound came out. Sheer terror washed over me and my whole body started shaking. I knew, at that moment, I would just lie there mute while I was raped and brutalised by – my dressing gown!

The terror this morning came from something a bit more substantial. The first incident wasn't too serious and has probably happened to many others. We had purchased new bedroom furniture before leaving on our trip to Victoria, and this morning I decided to organise the delivery. I rang the warehouse but the number was engaged, and although I kept trying every fifteen minutes or so over the course of the morning, it was constantly engaged. Several times I double checked the telephone number on the store docket but was confident I had not misdialled. It was close to lunchtime and I was almost ready to forget the whole thing and try again tomorrow, when I realised the number I had been calling was the one listed under 'Customer Contact' on the docket – my own number!

Taken as a single incident, this may not have worried me, and in fact I could even hear myself relating this story to friends and laughing about it. But as the day went forward, my mind seemed to travel in reverse.

For many years, I have been in the habit of tackling the crosswords in the newspaper and believe it's good for mental stimulation. But this morning, when I opened the paper and attempted what is considered the easiest one, I couldn't come up with a single answer. And not only that – I couldn't understand how crosswords worked! Ten minutes later I was still sitting with pen poised and nothing written.

'Don't panic,' I told myself. 'Do something else – some-thing you enjoy which involves no stress.'

I needed to hear my dear friend's voice – the voice of sanity – she'd know what to say and we'd end up laughing it off. I punched the Dial button on the handset to access the phone book, and paused. I could see her face, hear her voice but couldn't remember her name. I scrolled through the contact list, hoping her name would leap out at me, but I didn't recognise anyone, let alone her.

I started shaking. What was happening to me? Was this the onset of dementia – oh no, please God, anything but that. I had watched my mother struggle with this cruel disease, and the one real fear I harboured was that it might be hereditary. And it wasn't really the effect it would have on me. The sufferer gets past the stage where they know something is wrong and they withdraw into their own world. And in my mother's case, judging from her smiling countenance most days, that world seemed really pleasant. No, it was more the impact it would have on the people closest to me.

I put my head on the table and sobbed. Not even when I was diagnosed with cancer did I feel this scared. My first reaction when I need help is to reach out to HoN, but how could I ring him at work and what would I say? 'Hi, darl, guess what? I think I've lost my mind!' What did I expect him to do– send out a search party?

Fortunately, I had an appointment with my wonderful witch

later in the day. She'd know what to do, if only I could hang on till then. I suddenly understood why a wounded animal seeks the shelter of their burrow or nest, as I climbed into bed and waited out the time till I left home for the doctor's rooms.

By the time I met HoN at the oncologists a few hours later, I had painted on my Eleanor Rigby smile (the one I kept in a jar by the door), and steered the conversation towards general topics. Then I looked up and my doctor was walking towards me with a smile on her face. This was the first time she had seen me since my stay in Geelong Hospital and she wrapped me in a warm hug.

'We weren't sure we were going to see you again. You've certainly given us all a fright,' she said, and the smile disappeared. 'Apparently you had a look at the other side but, thankfully, decided to come back to us.'

This was news to me! I didn't remember seeing any white light at the end of a tunnel that I was being dragged towards. But then I suddenly remembered a strange incident I found hard to explain.

It was about the third day I had been in intensive care and I was lying with my eyes closed, when I felt someone grasp my hand. I opened my eyes but there was no one there, but suddenly 'the hand' started stroking mine in a very distinctive manner.

When my father had been in the hospice, I had sat with him every day for the last few weeks of his life. Often he was too weak for words, but we always maintained hand contact, and his way of showing his love was this particular way of stroking my hand. And at that moment, I knew my dad had come to help me.

'I'm going to get through this, Dad – I know you're watching over me,' I said, in my mind, 'but you know I'm strong, so please don't worry.'

Dad had 'visited' me once before, soon after his death. He had always owned a piano –he and Mum bought one even before purchasing their bed – and music was a big part of our family life. When Dad died, I found it sad that his piano stood abandoned, so I would go over to Mum's unit every few weeks and tickle the ivories in my amateurish manner.

This day Mum had gone shopping, so I was by myself. I started playing my favourite piece and, as often happened, I made several errors. But instead of skipping over these as I usually did, I went back to the beginning of the piece, started again and this time, played without any mistakes. Just as I hit the final chord, I felt a hand rest on my right shoulder, and Dad's voice came through very clearly.

'That's much better, dear,' he said.

I froze. I didn't know what to do. But one thing I was sure of. I did not want to turn round and see Dad standing there – I wouldn't be able to cope with it emotionally. So I closed the piano lid, picked up my bag and walked backwards to the front door. It was only as I stepped out on the porch that the heavy feeling surrounding me seemed to lift.

I often regretted this reaction and wondered how I would have felt looking into my dear dad's face again. Had I disappointed him? Was this why I hadn't seen or heard from him since?

And now, years later, he was visiting me again. But maybe this time, he was there to guide me through the next stage of my journey, and I just didn't recognise (or accept) that it was over. It certainly gives me a different perspective on death. How could it be frightening if your transition from one world to another is by the side of a loved one?

'So how have you been coping since you got back?' My doctor's question brought me back to the present.

'OK, I guess…I'm not…I don't…,' I said, and stopped.

HoN reached for my hand as I tried to blink away tears and suddenly I could no longer pretend. The morning's distress came spilling out of me.

Dr Tabitha listened quietly as I outlined why I was sure I had lost my mind. But then she alleviated my worries. 'You know you've had a very serious illness, and this can affect your whole body, including your mind. What you're experiencing is perfectly natural and is not permanent.'

She went on to explain in detail how the physical can affect the psychological, but that was enough for me. I didn't have dementia – that's all I needed to know!

But then she was talking about the chemotherapy and the effect it had had on my body. It was obvious she felt a responsibility for recommending a drug which had attacked my system so harshly.

It's mentioned as one of the rare side effects – the statistics are something like one in ten thousand people who might be affected – and these side effects were certainly pointed out to us.

From the moment we met my oncologist, we felt this woman had certainly chosen the right profession. Her understanding, empathy and ability to answer our questions in an easy to understand manner were traits we admired. I was anxious she should feel no responsibility.

'None of us ever think we're going to be that rare case, Tab,' I said, smiling to assure her. 'We had all the literature about every drug I'd be taking, and I knew the side effects. So, please, don't take this on yourself.'

She returned my smile, but I didn't feel she was convinced. What a pity, when she had just put my own mind to rest. Why couldn't I do the same for her?

Friday 14 March

Time to get the focus off cancer and concentrate on the heart. I've decided it's not as depressing as it sounds – having two health issues at the one time. That way you don't get too fixated on one or the other. It was to be my first meeting with a cardiologist (yet another 'gist' I hoped I'd never put 'my' in front of) and I had my list of questions ready.

When I was diagnosed with breast cancer, I nearly drowned in the information I was given regarding this condition. But although the doctors at Geelong Hospital had told me I had a heart condition called dilated cardiomyopathy, brought on by one of the chemotherapy drugs, I didn't know much more about it except that it really knocked you around. Well it certainly hadn't been too kind to me. When the oncologist at Geelong Hospital contacted Wonderful Witch to consult with her over my treatment, his opening words were 'I have one of your palliative care patients here.'

From the moment we sat down in the cardiologist's office, it was apparent the appointment had been squeezed in at the last minute. And as we had been sitting in the waiting room for forty-five minutes, we could only assume he was also running behind on his patient timetable.

We sat quietly while he read the report from the Geelong Hospital, then he confirmed the condition was indeed dilated cardiomyopathy, and said it could be treated with medication. After taking my blood pressure and commenting how low it was, he said that, because of this, he would have to be careful which medication he prescribed.

When I asked if this condition would affect my lifestyle, he muttered a few medical terms and surreptitiously consulted his watch. I tried a few more questions but the picture was clear – here is your prescription, now go and take your drugs. We were dismissed ten minutes later and as we made our way back to the car, HoN turned to me.

'Don't worry, babe,' he said, with an encouraging smile. 'There are plenty more cardiologists around and it's important we find one you can relate to. Sounds as if it will be an ongoing situation for the rest of your life.'

Yes, it made sense, but when we arrived home, my frustration level was at a peak. Bleeding hell! What was I in for? Did it shorten my life? Would my heart eventually recover? How long would I need medication? Did this make me susceptible to a heart attack? I realised how little I knew, and this was not a position I was comfortable with.

I headed to the study, sat down at the computer and clicked on the Google engine. But just before I accessed one of the many, many sights devoted to this particular heart condition, I could suddenly hear my mother's words about families who constantly referred to medical dictionaries back in the 1950s.

'No good can come of that,' she'd say. 'Leaves itself open to misdiagnosis and you'll always remember the worst thing.'

What the heck – I needed to know. But I didn't realise the importance of Mum's wise words until I typed in the words 'dilated cardiomyopathy' and wished I hadn't!

> About 70% of people die within five years of when their symptoms begin and the prognosis worsens as the heart becomes more dilated and functions less well.

I was so gobsmacked by this piece of information, the shabby sentence structure didn't even faze me. And there was even more doom and gloom.

> About 50% of deaths are sudden probably resulting from an abnormal heart rhythm.
>
> The decreased heart function can affect the lungs, liver and other body systems.

This wasn't answering my questions, just posing more. I switched the computer off and stared at the blank screen. The sooner we found another cardiologist, the better.

Tuesday 8 April

I've promised my oncologist I'll discuss radiotherapy with a specialist she has recommended and 'discuss' is the operative word. You see, I'm not really sure I want to go ahead with it. When I first started this whole medical journey, and accepted I would need some pretty intensive treatment to get rid of the cancer, my main thought was 'Let's just get on with it.' But now that one of the treatments, a chemotherapy drug, has permanently damaged my heart, I'm scared about bombarding my body with rays? And this radiotherapy will be given in close proximity to my already damaged heart. No, I think they'll have their work cut out convincing me that this is a good thing!

Wonderful Wicked Witch pointed out that treatment for my particular cancer usually comprises thirty radiotherapy treatments, necessitating a visit to the clinic every day from Monday to Friday for six weeks. As I sat in the waiting room of the clinic this morning, I went over and over the reservations I had about this particular form of treatment and also the tedium of the whole regime. And then we were being ushered into the doctor's office.

The radiation oncologist was a quietly spoken South African woman in her early sixties, who had a beautifully gentle manner and the kindest eyes. She started to discuss how radiation treatment was one more factor in fighting my cancer, but I didn't want to waste her valuable time.

'I'm sorry, but I'm only here because I promised my oncologist I would see you, but I don't really want this.'

I paused, but she just sat quietly, waiting for me to elaborate.

'I've already had damage to the heart through treatment and because the radiation will be directed onto my left breast, this is a bit too close for comfort for me. I just don't want to risk it.'

She leant forward and her eyes softened even more. 'I can understand your reluctance, but there are safeguards we can use. Also, radiotherapy is a very precise science and a lot of care is taken to pinpoint the exact spot where it's needed so there's no risk to surrounding areas.'

I still wasn't convinced, and was trying to formulate my next question, when HoN spoke up.

'What are the statistics we're looking at?' he asked, and I smiled a 'thank you' for his logical mind. 'What are the odds of the cancer coming back if we don't have radiotherapy?' he added.

I smiled. If 'we' don't have radiotherapy? How sweet! He's going to join me every day, is he? He really was going through every step with me, and I sent him a hug through my eyes.

'If you go ahead with radiotherapy,' the doctor said, 'there's only a two per cent chance of the cancer recurring. If you don't have it, then those odds go up to thirty per cent.'

We were silent as her words impacted on us. Our surprised expressions mirrored each other. No wonder my witch had insisted we keep this appointment.

'Is there no other way I can reduce the risks of cancer coming back?' I asked.

'Only if you had a complete mastectomy,' she replied. 'Then your odds would be back to two per cent.'

This was a fairly drastic resolution and it did surprise me when I didn't rule this option out immediately. But hey, I already had an imperfect pair, with half of one breast gone. Instead of Won Hung Loh and Won Satay (Sat High!) I could have a double mastectomy, a breast reduction, and attain the pert little boobs I had always dreamt of.

The doctor leant forward and touched my knee. 'I realise you'll need to give this some thought, but if you decide to go ahead with the radiotherapy, we should do it within the next few weeks. I'll take you round to the technicians and they can do your mark-up, so they have the details if you decide to proceed.'

I spent the next half hour lying very still while a couple of young girls hovered over me with a black felt pen. They talked about 'tattooing' me so the machine would know exactly where to direct the radiotherapy, but laughed when I asked for a dolphin.

'I'm afraid we only deal in full stops,' one said, as she placed a precise dot on the side of my left breast.

'Doesn't matter,' I thought. 'I'll be putting a full stop to this whole thing soon anyway.' The option of the mastectomy was looking more and more attractive. I walked out of the radiotherapy clinic, glad this would be my first and final visit.

Thursday 10 April

It's been a little over twenty-four hours since I had the discussion about radiotherapy with Dr Anna, the radiology oncologist, and I'm still undecided which track I should go down – the one which leads to radiotherapy or the one which veers off to a mastectomy. Those statistics she quoted keep going round in my head as the one fear I do have is that the cancer may return. And if it does, I can't fight it with chemotherapy any more. I've discussed the options with HoN, but for once, it didn't seem to help.

'When you think about it, radiation's only six weeks of feeling like shit,' he said. 'That'll fly by and it'll be over before you know it.'

Well, guess what? I don't want to feel like shit for six hours let alone six weeks.

Although I haven't had chemotherapy since mid-February, I still remember what 'feeling like shit' is all about, and two months later the toxins are still leaching out of my body. My toenails and fingernails are discoloured, the skin on my feet is peeling and my toes, fingers and tongue are still numb. Why would I want to expose any more of my body to treatment?

Yes, at this stage, mastectomy is looking like a pretty good option. And I never thought I'd hear myself say that! But then my world swings even further off its axis and my own health problems take a back seat.

My big brother, who has always been my rock, is ringing to tell me he's been diagnosed with prostate cancer. My stomach starts churning. I thought I could cope with anything – anything but this. I grasp on to a thread when I remember he has been very careful about regular checkups. Dad had prostate cancer and Chris is aware of the genetic link. I listen as he explains about PSA levels and try to pick up on how he is coping with the news. He sounds fine, but then he always does. I suspect it's that whole 'protective' thing big brothers seem to have with their little sisters. The doctor has explained the treatment options which are available, but I can't take it all on board.

After I hang up, I allow the tears to come. I'm suddenly scared I am going to lose him and that thought terrifies me, even more than my own cancer diagnosis. The phone conversation seems a blur – I hope I said all the right things. But what am I talking about? What 'right things'? I can never remember thinking 'Well, they didn't say the right thing' after telling friends and relatives of my diagnosis. I guess we all feel inadequate at times when we search for something to say which won't sound trite or cliché. But we shouldn't. Having been the recipient of phone calls, text messages, letters, emails and cards, there was not one 'wrong' word amongst them – just an overwhelming feeling of support from everyone. It's at times like this I wished my brother didn't live in Sydney or that I didn't live in Adelaide. I desperately need to give him a reassuring hug – and maybe get one back.

I don't really use the phrase 'I'll send out positive thoughts for you' any more. I used to say it all the time, but it can sound a bit trite – cliché, even. I don't use the phrase but I do practise it and have great faith in its strength. So I sit quietly in the lounge, which has always been my 'sacred place' with its soft pastel colours and the muted ticking of the marble clock, I concentrate so hard on my brother's face thousands of kilometres away, I can even see the cancer leaving his body. Suddenly the decision regarding my radiotherapy seems unimportant.

Tuesday 15 April

Don't ask me how it works, but I've always believed that people carry the traits peculiar to the star sign they are born under. My Taurean man can be as stubborn as all come-out, my Leo son commands centre stage whenever we're together and my Cancerian friend is a creative nurturer. As a Libran, I tend to see both sides of an argument, which sounds great, but I've never thought of this as a positive. You see, there are times when I can't make a bloody decision to save myself, and this latest dilemma is a screaming example of that!

Radiotherapy versus mastectomy – I've even made a list of all the pros and cons – and they're all beautifully balanced. Well, they have to be, don't they, because that's what Librans do! Fortunately my regular appointment with Wonderful Wicked was due this morning and I was hoping she could perhaps clarify the options a bit more. Well, all right, I'll be honest – I really wanted her to make the decision for me.

As we take a seat in her office, she asks how we went with Dr Anna, the radiology oncologist.

'She's such a lovely person,' I said, 'and explained things really well.' I paused. 'But I'm still not certain whether to have radiotherapy. I still have trepidation about the danger to my heart – that's had enough damage done to it.'

As soon as I utter those words, I realise how insensitive I was being. I knew no matter what I said, this wonderful doctor would always harbour some guilt about the adverse reaction I had had to one of the chemotherapy drugs she recommended.

'But I know it's not that simple, Tab, and here's where I need your help. We were told the chances of the cancer returning are only two per cent if I have the radiotherapy and thirty per cent if I don't. The only other alternative is to have a complete mastectomy, and my odds would stay at two per cent.'

I was well aware I was probably telling my doctor how to suck eggs, but hey, I do have a rather bad habit of stating the bleeding obvious at times.

She looked at me for a few seconds, and then shook her head. 'I'm so sorry, Claire, I'm afraid an operation's out of the question at this stage. An anaesthetist wouldn't give you a general anaesthetic with your heart being as it is.'

And there it was! The decision had been taken out of my hands. Wasn't that what I wanted?

HoN reached out and grabbed my hand, realising what a body blow this was for me. At least he was wise enough not to repeat his earlier words, 'It's only six more weeks of feeling like shit.'

As a wave of nausea swept over me, I suddenly realised I had already made up my mind which route I wanted to travel. I wanted a mastectomy. And it wasn't because that option had suddenly been taken away. These boobs of mine had been a millstone I had carried round all my life and I could never ignore them. When I was younger, I was forced to buy clothes one size larger than I needed just to accommodate them. And during my teenage dating years, I had to sometimes remind guys just where my eyes were located. As I reached maturity (well, okay, I put on weight) my bras resembled slingshots large enough to defend Windsor Castle! And let's not even talk about my shoulders, where years of carrying the twins around had left ruts deep enough to bury the entire potato crop of Ireland. And that was just the vanity angle!

My mind flew back to the day of the cancer diagnosis, and lying on the table while the doctor ran the ultrasound over each breast. There was a pretty intensive concentration on the left breast, where the cancer was eventually found, but the doctor did say initially that there was a suspicious area in the right breast as well. After a lot of examining the area, he dismissed it and gave the OK on the right breast, but I knew I couldn't bear to go through all that again.

And one more thing I had to consider as well. If the cancer did come back, chemotherapy would be out of the question, so what would I fight it with?

Yes, I wanted a mastectomy more than I realised, but bugger, bugger, bugger – it wasn't to be.

Sunday 20 April

My emotions have been all over the place the past five days since hearing a mastectomy is out of the question. Radiotherapy is now my only option if I want to ensure the cancer doesn't return. The over-riding emotion when I arrived home from the doctor's was one of depression. I really didn't want to go through six weeks of treatment, every Monday to Friday, and even though Dr Anna had told me there would be no danger to my heart, I wasn't completely convinced.

Then my depression turned to anger. Why didn't the breast surgeon give me the option of a double mastectomy when I was originally diagnosed? Even as I had this thought, I could see how ridiculous this sounded. What surgeon would suggest removing a perfectly healthy breast – one in which there was no sign of cancer? Oh well, it's too late now – I just need to get my mind onto something else. And so the constantly changing landscape of my hair and head now took centre stage.

For several weeks I've been displaying what can only be described as bum fluff all over my head – certainly bum fluff that's lost its sense of direction! I had been told by several people that when your hair does come back, it can be an entirely different colour. Wow! Maybe I'll get fuchsia! But apparently the message didn't get through, because what I can see now is almost black.

This was so much of a shock that I was unable to walk past a mirror without stopping and staring at my black fuzz. Since my early teenage years, I had been a blonde (with the help of the lemon tree initially and the bottle ever after) and this totally new colour was hard to get used to. And then I remembered the lock of pitch-black hair wrapped in a piece of cellophane which

Mum had taped in my baby book after my very first haircut. It didn't stay that colour for long, as I reverted to white blonde as a toddler.

I was telling a friend about my new crop and she related the story of a woman she knew who, before breast cancer, had always dyed her mousy brown hair a soft blonde, but when her post-chemo hair grew back, it was steel grey. Determined to get her identity back as soon as possible, she headed off to the hairdresser and requested her usual blonde.

'You'll have to find someone else to do it,' the hairdresser said. 'I think you look stunning with grey hair, so I'm not going to change it.'

I told my friend that if my post-chemo mop turned steel grey and a hairdresser refused to change it, then she'd still be trying to extract her straightening wand from a distant place one year later!

No, I was very close to a visit to my girl to get the black fuzz altered, and while it was so short, perhaps a nice nut brown would do the trick.

Friday 25 April

'If it was going to improve, it should have by now,' the cardiologist said.

My heart sank, just to reinforce the message. I was hoping my ejection fraction would have a higher reading, but it hadn't improved much at all. Yes, we found another cardiologist, although I can't say he's someone I warm to. He didn't do himself any favours when he chose to take a private phone call during my appointment. The call was from the headmaster of a private college he was desperate to get his children into. Anyway, back to the ejection fraction.

I've never been one for numbers. Maths bored me to death at school, and any mention of fractions meant friction when the teacher singled me out to supply the answer. But since my heart has decided to play up, I needed to accept that an ejection fraction is a mathematical figure I should not ignore.

The ventricular ejection fraction is the fraction of blood pumped out of a ventricle with each heart beat. A healthy heart has a fraction of approximately sixty per cent, and when I was in hospital in Geelong, mine was down to twenty-five per cent. At a test conducted a few weeks after I arrived home, the fraction had risen to thirty-seven per cent and the latest one was thirty-eight per cent. Because the number was increasing each time, I was feeling optimistic. The cardiologist was expecting a bigger improvement. But the number had stayed the same.

It's fine to tell people to have a positive outlook, but sometimes you just can't be bothered, particularly when you hear the constant splash of water as your glass half-full is knocked over yet again.

Looking back over the last ten months, I sometimes felt I was drowning. When I discovered the lump, I was fairly confident it was yet another benign cyst. After all, hadn't I already had two removed years ago? And the doctor did warn me there would probably be others.

Sorry, it's cancer.

All right, I have cancer, but it's a very small lump. I had a mammogram only eight months ago, so I'm feeling confident it is confined to the breast.

Grade II cancer has been found in one of the fourteen lymph nodes taken – we'll have to take a larger sample.

In a matter of only two weeks, I heard of two acquaintances who needed only radiotherapy after their operations. I began to think there would be three of us.

You will need the whole compilation treatment.

I was feeling confident that I would sail through chemotherapy – after all, doesn't everyone tell me I look so well!

You're one of the very rare people who have experienced an adverse reaction to one of the drugs. Unfortunately it has permanently affected your heart.

Can't bear the idea of six weeks of radiotherapy, and after finding out a mastectomy would give me the same low odds of the cancer returning, am leaning towards the latter.

An anaesthetist would be reluctant to approve an operation because your heart is not strong enough.

Yes, I really should have changed my appointment date with the cardiologist, because guess what – it's another bloody Friday!

Monday 28 April

I started radiation treatment today. The first day in the 'six weeks of feeling like shit'! But I'm actually pleased it's finally here. The way I see it, the sooner I start, the sooner I finish. The clinic I've chosen to have my treatment at is not necessarily the one closest to home, but it is the one I feel more comfortable with.

As I sat in the waiting room, I noticed other patients greeting each other like old friends. I guess with daily appointments for five or six weeks, you are bound to see the same faces and build up a feeling of camaraderie. A woman sitting opposite started to discuss the weather with me – making the new girl feel welcome, I guess – but my name was called before I could continue the conversation.

The technician took me through to a change area and pointed to a locker with my name on it. 'That's where you leave your gown after each treatment,' she said, and then smiled, 'except on the final day when you can bin it.'

She looked quite thrilled at the prospect as she pointed to a receptacle in the corner, but I was finding it hard to match her enthusiasm. Maybe you had to actually do it – bin it, that is – to experience the euphoria, because my 'bin there, done that' day seemed too far away at this stage. And then I was ushered into a minuscule changing room and told to remove all clothing from the top half.

Easy for them to say, because as I lifted my arms, my elbow hit a small shelf and a box of tissues hit the floor. Luckily the bottles on the shelf remained upright. One bottle held what looked like baby oil and that was to help remove the black felt pen marks they used to measure you up. The other bottle contained moisturising lotion. I had been told that radiotherapy was similar to sunburn, with redness, drying and eventual peeling of the skin.

'Better remember to do both sides,' I thought, 'otherwise Cat's Arse will be smooth and moist and Wun Hung Loh, dry and withered.'

As soon as I emerged from my cubicle, two technicians led me into a room and helped me up onto a cold steel table with a large machine hovering above. They chatted as they measured where the radiotherapy would be directed, and explained that because it is such a precise science, they would always have two people checking the measurements. And then I was by myself in the room.

My ears picked up on the faint strains of music from a radio station, but my eyes were fixated on the machine overhead. Suddenly there was a loud click and then the buzz as the treatment started. I willed myself to lie perfectly still. They had measured me up lying exactly here, and not a fraction of a centimetre to the left or right.

What happens if I sneeze? Oh no, my nose was itching. Would I be zapped in the wrong place? Does it matter how deeply I breathe? Hang on – I still had questions. My eyes roamed around the room but this time, there wasn't even a boring poster to distract me. Somebody had affixed stickers to the machine, but they were the sort given to children for good work at kindergarten. I started devising my own set of stickers. After all, if you have to stare at this thing every day for the next six weeks, you may as well try and find some humour.

> This machine is operated by aliens who have now drained your brain of any intelligence. That's why it didn't take long!
>
> Or maybe
>
> Think of this as a tropical holiday – you'll certainly come home with a suntan!

I was just composing a third sticker when the buzzing stopped. I had been warned not to move when this happened as there was still an additional short zap to be applied in this area.

When it stopped, the technicians came back into the room.

'Well done,' one of the girls said. 'Only one more to go.' She repositioned the machine and left the room once more.

Click, bzz. I started counting. 1 and 2 and 3 and 4 and… I reached 42 before it stopped. I wondered if it was going to be the same number each day. At least that would keep my mind occupied instead of worrying about involuntary reactions from my nasal passages, or any other orifice!

Back in the cubicle, I took my gown off and examined my left breast but it looked exactly the same as it did when I arrived. I put some oil on a tissue and wiped off the black pen marks, and wondered what the technicians would say if, before the next treatment, I drew a furry tail extending from my cat's arse! Smiling at the thought, I whacked on some moisturiser, got dressed and walked through to Reception. How easy was that!

Friday 9 May

One of the things Delores D'Lump can lay claim to is that she was a HER-2 positive early stage breast cancer (and believe me, she was chuffed when I told her). This occurs in fifteen to twenty per cent of breast cancer cases, and when you have this tag, part of the treatment recommended can be Herceptin. This drug is administered intravenously every week for a period of twelve months and I had already received eight doses of Herceptin before I left for my holiday.

Although this drug is considered to be a breakthrough in the treatment of some cancers (and certainly Wonderful Wicked was excited I would be given this option to fight my particular cancer) one of the less common side effects is the possibility it will damage your heart. Even before you start treatment, it is recommended you have an echocardiogram or MUGA, a multigated blood pool imaging scan to check how well your heart is functioning. The damage to my heart however, had been caused by one of the chemotherapy drugs, Doxorubicin, and because of this, further chemo treatment was ceased. But Witch still held out hope that I could continue with Herceptin.

Given that the possibility of heart damage was mentioned in every reference to Herceptin, it may be hard to understand why I didn't just write it off as a treatment option. But one thing which was niggling away at the back of my mind was the fact I had not completed my full chemotherapy cycle, therefore the cancer still might be in my system. And that thought terrified me!

I had been discussing this with HoN over the past few weeks, trying to make a decision, but once again the Libran scales refused to swing either way. And then suddenly this morning, soon after waking up, I had a 'light bulb' moment. There was no doubt in my mind any more, and I felt confident with my decision, as I sat in the oncologist's room.

'I've weighed up the possible adverse affects, Tab,' I said, leaning forward in my chair, 'and that includes the possibility of damage to my heart, but hey, that's already happened, hasn't it? No, I've decided I want to take out this extra insurance to stop the cancer recurring, so when can we get started?'

I sat back and waited for her reaction. Why wasn't she smiling and agreeing with me? After all, this was the part of my treatment she was most eager about – I wanted her to be pleased with my decision.

'I'm so sorry, Clare,' she said, and frowned. 'I'm afraid it's no longer an option. You see, the government wouldn't approve funding for you to use Herceptin with your heart condition. Unfortunately your ejection fraction's too low.' She went on to explain that it costs the government $50,000 per annum per patient to be treated with Herceptin and they use the ejection fraction as a guideline for suitability.

Shit! I had that awful sinking feeling in my stomach I used to get at school when I sat for a test and only just missed passing by a couple of marks. My disappointment was reflected on my doctor's face as I realised the news was just as devastating for her – Herceptin was her baby. She had so much faith in the drug and really wanted me to be able to take it. But sadly, I also saw a flash of guilt in her eyes. When was she going to stop blaming herself?

Wednesday 4 June

From the minute I got out of bed this morning, I've been running on red cordial. I've already done two loads of washing, cleaned the kitchen, re-organised my wardrobe and cleared my emails – and it's only nine a.m.! I'm trying to keep my mind away from health problems, not mine but my brother's. Since he was diagnosed with prostate cancer two months ago, he has been meeting with the specialist and weighing up treatment options available. And today he goes into hospital for a prostatectomy.

I don't know what's going on with our family recently. My cousin (my brother from another mother) was diagnosed with prostate cancer a few months before my breast cancer diagnosis. Because we work together, I had been able to follow each step of his treatment, a treatment called Brachytherapy This necessitated an operation where the doctor planted radioactive 'seeds' next to the prostate and the seeds target that area only.

Comparing this treatment with what they were recommending for me, I was quite envious. How simple is that? Just one trip to hospital, one operation and get on with your life. I was conveniently ignoring the fact that every treatment has side effects, and he had his fair share. And now it was my brother's turn – in for his operation and, hopefully, no further treatment.

It seemed so much simpler to have 'bloke's cancer', although I did get a different perspective on that just recently. One of our bookshops had a week where they were promoting local authors and I was discussing writing with a gentleman who bought my books.

'Are you working on anything at the moment?' he asked.

I nodded. 'Yes, I'm writing about my experience with breast cancer.'

'Should be writing one about prostate cancer,' he stated, ducking his head and peering over his glasses. 'There're too many men with it these days.' He shook his head. 'But of course that isn't the sexy cancer to have.'

I was rather taken aback by this comment. Not once has the thought 'Gee, glad I've got the sexy cancer' passed through my mind. Not that I was in any danger of getting the other! But it wasn't until I was lying in bed that night that I fully grasped what he was talking about with his strange use of that adjective.

The colour pink had become synonymous with breast cancer, with every second product emblazoned with a pink bow denoting the company would give part proceeds to the fight against this particular cancer. And high-profile people like Sarah O'Hare, Olivia Newton John, Jane McGrath and others were fighting the fight to raise more funds for research, and that kept the topic in the media constantly. The only time you heard about prostate cancer was when a television or sporting identity was diagnosed, but then it would fade into the background once again. Where were their coloured ribbon symbol and their ongoing stories?

Perhaps I could take up the baton for all those men out there who have been diagnosed, and make this the subject of my next book. If I have to start somewhere, I only need look at my own family, where my father, brother and cousin were all diagnosed with this 'unsexy' cancer. And they all chose different treatments.

Thinking of my brother suddenly drags me back to the present. This day seems to be going on endlessly while I wait for news of his operation. I should have set myself a project – something which would consume my brain, blocking out any opportunity to think about cancer – or operations – or brothers. Once again, I feel the tyranny of the physical distance between us and wonder if it would have been easier being in Sydney waiting for the news with my sister in law and niece, two other women who think he's pretty special. But then the phone is ringing and the smile nearly splits my face as I hear my brother's voice, albeit a bit slurred.

'Hi, little sis, it's over – went well. Knew you'd need to hear my voice before you were convinced I was OK.'

Suddenly, everything was right with my world. The tears that come after I hang up are tears of relief this time.

Friday 6 June

That's it – it's all over! I had my final radiation treatment this morning. Let's hope those bzzes have done their work.

It's certainly intense, every day Monday to Friday for six weeks, and becomes a new way of life, and in a strange way, I'm going to miss it (something I thought I'd never hear myself say). Don't get me wrong – I won't miss the tiresome trip there and back each day, and I certainly won't miss the bleeding great machine hovering over my left breast. In the end, I didn't get around to making a special sticker for the machine, to brighten up the next patient's day. The best I could find in the shop this morning on the way to treatment was a sticker that declared 'I DID IT', which pretty much sums it up anyway

No, it's the people I dealt with at the clinic – the gorgeous technicians who 'give us this day our daily dose' – my radio fairies, as I called them. We've shared details of families, favourite television programs, fashion and movies and now I won't see them again, or at least I hope not!

Yesterday, they asked if I wanted them to wear anything special for my last treatment. I was touched that they would bother making a celebration of the last radiotherapy treatment, but couldn't come up with anything creative on the spur of the moment, so reached for the breast cancer badge.

'Let's all wear something pink,' I said, mentally going through my wardrobe and knowing this wouldn't be too difficult a task for me.

And when one of my radio fairies came to collect me from the reception area this morning, I burst out laughing, along with several other patients waiting for treatment. She had donned a pair of her daughter's pink fairy wings, had a tiara perched on the top of her head and was waving a magic wand. The other 'fairy' joined us and smiled at me under a bright pink headscarf, and with my pink parka and matching scarf, we could have formed a group. The Three 'Musk'eteers maybe?

And the celebration was not just restricted to our clothing. I was told to bring a favourite CD to play during treatment. In retrospect, I should have opted for something like Il Divo, because the whole idea of the treatment is to stay perfectly still – a task I found almost impossible to obey as I listened to the throbbing beat of the Rogue Traders with Nat Bassingthwaite belting out the lyrics of 'Voodoo Child'.

I've just arrived home and I have to admit I feel a bit flat, which is strange. Initially I was against having this treatment and reluctantly accepted the fait accompli. But then I realise it's really nothing to do with the treatment. It's the realisation that as we go through life, we meet people who make an indelible impression upon us. But because of the nature of the contact, these dealings can be fleeting, and once the need has been met, there is no reason to continue the relationship. These wonderful techs helped me through yet one more stage of my recovery – I hope my thanks were adequate.

Sunday 22 June

We had decided on a quiet Sunday; one of those lazy days where you accept that nothing much will get done and it's not going to bother you. I was relishing having a new Jeffery Deaver book to devour and had put on a Norah Jones CD in the background. HoN was watching sport on TV, with the sound on mute, so we were both happy in our own worlds. I don't know what made me look up at the television – maybe it was the movement of the words running across the bottom of the screen – but suddenly I was riveted to the newsflash.

> Jane McGrath, cancer campaigner and wife of cricketer Glenn McGrath, has died of breast cancer.

I felt as though I'd been hit in the stomach, the pain was so real. I doubled over and the television screen blurred. But hang on, why was I so shocked? We had all followed this woman's battle over the past few years, and the news the cancer was back several months ago had not been a good sign.

Yes, it was terribly sad that a young mother with a wonderful husband and beautiful family should leave them when there was so much more living to do. And hadn't she worked tirelessly making people aware of breast cancer and the need for money to fund more breast care nurses? It wasn't as if I knew her personally. But none of this seemed to matter, because I'd forgotten where my tears-off tap was located, as my eyes were drawn back to those running words.

But there was another emotion which was just as strong, and that was one of fear. Oh my God, had it only just dawned on me? That people actually die of cancer! Yes, it sounds a classic case of stating the bleeding obvious once again. But when you're diagnosed with something which still scares the bejesus out of most of us, you can't afford to dwell on that aspect for even a few moments. I'd only had one instant since diagnosis that I could recall where I'd actually played out the 'what ifs' in my head.

Although my tears were silent, HoN and his sensitive radar was still able to pick up on my distress, and wrapped me in a hug. But I knew I couldn't share my fear – the real reason for my tears – it just wouldn't be fair. He'd worked so hard concentrating on the positives. How could I undo all that good work with this ghastly negativity I felt?

'Those poor children,' I said, 'losing their beautiful mother.'

HoN nodded.

It was headlines again on the evening news, but I had something else, anything else to do away from the television, and soon the emotion of the day caught up with me and I headed for bed. My bones were aching and my skin even felt sensitive and I realised how much I'd been hung out to dry emotionally. Sleep would be a saviour. But an hour and a half later, I was still wide awake and the tears were making an uncomfortable pillow.

This day, 22 June, is one of the most difficult days to get through each year. It's my son's birthday – the son who has alienated himself from me and I'm not even sure why – and I had just gone through yet another year when I had not seen his beautiful face and hugged him tight.

Friday 25 July

It should be a relief that all the treatment for my cancer is finished. And even though the chemotherapy had to be cut short, and the added insurance of Herceptin was not an option in the end, I will continue the daily hormone pill, which gives me aching joints, hot flushes, thinning hair and weight gain (fantastic!) and try to believe we have done enough.

The heart situation is not quite as simple. Initially I was focused on this mysterious ejection fraction the doctors talked about, and it became a challenge to see how much my magic number could improve. But now I have accepted it's not so much a matter of my heart healing completely (apparently that's not going to happen), but more an improvement in the quality of my life through medication.

Due to the ongoing relationship with my cardiologist, it was important I find someone who could answer my questions and whom I felt comfortable with – I needed a cardiologist with heart – and that's how I think of the doctor I see now. Right from the moment he shook my hand, I took to this man with his calm demeanour and eyes that disappear into his smile. He shares a surname with the famous Walt and I have named him MMM (Marvellous Mickey Mouse). HoN has his own names for my oncologist WWW and cardiologist MMM – he calls them Stalactite and Stalagmite and I had to admit I could see his point!

When I was first diagnosed, one of the people I felt a desperate need to talk to was my mother and I guess that's perfectly natural. No matter how old you are, there will always be situations where you want to believe that a mother's kiss will make it all better. But over the course of this year, I have found my own substitute MOM and this is my 'Mattress of Medicos' I constantly collapsed back upon. Whether it was 'deer' doe-eyed Sophie, the clinical nurse answering questions regarding side effects of chemotherapy, Jane the beautiful breast care nurse 'I mean it, Claire, ring me any time of the day or night' or my JOI (Jackpot of Ists) oncologist, radiologist, cardiologist, psychiatrist, who all showed remarkable patience and understanding, the support has always been there.

If someone had asked me a year ago how I would be feeling at the end of my treatment, I probably would have replied 'Bloody relieved.' But it's weird; there's not the euphoria I thought there would be. Now that I can catch up with people who don't necessarily hold a medical degree, I feel the threads linking me to my support team growing thinner and stretching further away, and I'm scared. Maybe it's because my emotional reaction to situations has been anything but typical since this all started, and the doctors I've been dealing with have seen it all before, so any reaction is expected and accepted. But will my friends understand this?

Just the other day I arrived home after having lunch with a group of friends. As usual, we had spent the couple of hours laughing and joking, and my mood was high. But no sooner had I walked in the door, than I sat down at the dining room table, put my head in my hands and sobbed. How can my glass half full of hope turn so quickly into a glass half empty with despair?

But then perhaps it's the same reaction I had as a mother of young sons who, throughout their adventurous childhood, gave me several dramatic moments. At the moment of having to rush them to hospital, while keeping your cool, every mother seems to cope. It's only after the event, when you know your child is going to be all right, that you're able to give in to emotion. Maybe now I knew I was going to be all right, and everything that could be, had been done, my emotion could no longer be contained.

Sunday 31 August

It's a year to the day since my diagnosis – my 'year of living dangerously'. Just as well I didn't know what lay ahead of me as I sat in the doctor's surgery twelve months ago and heard those two words 'your cancer'. And perhaps it's a blessing I have never encouraged the psychic abilities which seem to have attached themselves to the female members of my mother's family.

My great grandmother, Grannie Mills, died well before I was born, but she was so admired and loved by the family, I felt I knew her. Apparently she was able to see people's auras, and her assessment of strangers was always proven to be spot on. My grandmother could remember her mother saying someone had a 'muddy' aura, which meant 'They're up to no good, lass.'

My maternal grandmother, Sabina Weeks, lived with our family until I was twelve years old and was part of my life well into my thirties. She had a particular talent with the art of psychometry, which is the ability to gain impressions of a person by holding an object that is special to that person, such as a piece of jewellery. Followers of this psychic ability believe the object brings forth images and mental thought forms, and a person able to do this can sense images of things without knowing anything about the object or the person it belongs to.

I was not averse to using Gran's special gift for my own convenience and would sometimes give her an object belonging to a new boyfriend to see if my prince had indeed come! I can remember one particular boyfriend having his cynicism quickly eradicated as I shared Gran's insight with him – details which I had been unaware of and proved quite unusual and one hundred per cent accurate.

And then there was my own mother. Throughout my

younger years, I often kidded myself I was one of the most popular girls at the local primary school because there were always requests from classmates to accompany me home each day. But I soon learnt it was not my sparkling personality or my irresistible magnetism. It was my mother's offer of afternoon tea and the reading of the tea leaves afterwards.

She would have the kettle boiling as we walked in the back door, and each girl's cup quickly drunk, tea leaves swirled around and the cup upended over the saucer in a matter of minutes. The most difficult task was the patience needed as we would be instructed to hold both hands on the cup as the vibrations penetrated. Several pairs of wide eyes would be riveted on my mother's face as she made predictions for my friends. Not surprisingly, these always included their dreams being fulfilled!

But this wasn't my mother's only psychic ability. Much to my constant embarrassment, she would stop and talk to perfect strangers, giving advice on what she 'saw'.

One day we were travelling on the bus into the city and she stood up and walked over to a woman a few seats away. 'I hope you don't mind me telling you this, dear,' she said, placing her hand on the woman's arm, 'but you must be careful around a garage door.'

The woman looked horrified, and I was already anticipating the driver stopping the bus, calling the authorities and dragging this mad woman and her daughter off the bus! But then I realised the look on the woman's face wasn't one of horror, but in fact, amazement.

'That is really strange,' she said. 'I don't usually take the bus to work, but this morning, when I went to back the car out of the garage, the door crashed down on the bonnet of my car.'

Mum breathed a sigh of relief. 'Thank goodness it's already happened and you're safe,' she said.

Those three matriarchs of our family have been out of my life for quite some time now, and maybe, in a way, that's a blessing. Perhaps they would have been tempted to look into the future and I would have been tempted to ask what they saw. Who knows? But I'm now convinced you're better coping with things as they happen rather than anticipating something you know you cannot change. I can look back and feel proud I've made it – that I came through the other side.

Often people say these situations can be life-changing, and in some ways they are. I can't honestly say that I'm suddenly appreciating life more because I have been doing that for some time. But I think that's a natural part of the ageing process. On my beach walks, I often stop and pick up a perfect shell and marvel at how clever nature is. And smile when I notice how a devoted dog looks at his owner. And I've always loved the start of a new day, when the world has been refreshed and there's potential for a new adventure. Yes, it sounds corny, doesn't it? But I don't care!

There are two things, however, which have changed – or have changed me. One of them is a 'don't sweat the small stuff' attitude. So many times I would worry about details which, in the big plan, didn't really matter. So what if the house is untidy and there's a knock at the door! So what, if this top doesn't exactly match those pants!

The second change is one of tolerance. Oh, don't get me wrong. I'm far from being angelic (a statement everyone who knows me will readily confirm!) but I'm not as critical of others as I have been in the past. I suddenly understood that we're all so fragile and, no matter how hard the shell, we all need some sort of understanding.

I'm still having my down times but fortunately they don't last too long. Yes, faced with your own mortality, life suddenly becomes valuable, and I really don't want to waste it being miserable. I have been told that when I was seriously ill in hospital in Victoria, I 'had a look at the other side', but decided to come back. Maybe there wasn't a whole lot over there to interest me. Or maybe they just weren't ready for me yet. I'll never know. But it's scared me enough not to persevere reading a book that doesn't grab me in the first few chapters (there's too many good books out there I still haven't read) and also to live by the following creed:

> Life's too short not to have your morning juice in a champagne glass full of dragonfly ice blocks.

Epilogue

When I penned those final words, I was blissfully unaware this saga would go on for yet another three years! You see, I'm writing this from the same hospital where I had Delores's coming-out party and recovering from yet another operation.

No, there hasn't been secondary cancer discovered, thank God! That's a fear that creeps into your thoughts when you least expect it. It doesn't take over your thinking, but it can give you a gentle nudge at certain times, especially the yearly mammogram. The medical term for secondary cancer is 'metastasis' but neither my thought processes nor my tongue can quite get around that word, so I just hope like hell the doctors never find that Delores has a little sister, Diandra! Anyway, back to the reason for this latest operation.

Throughout this experience (and please don't call it a 'journey'!), I have mentioned once (or two thousand times) how much grief I've endured over the years being landed with large breasts. And when it became necessary to take half the breast on the left side, I was left with such an uneven pair I was in danger of listing to the right each time I adopted an upright position! At last, here was my chance to not only 'even the score' but have a reduction so I could actually paint my toenails without hyperventilating!

But why the long wait, I hear you ask? (Or maybe you couldn't give a toss!) Well, with my particular heart condition, the cardiologist and anaesthetist had been reluctant to give me the go ahead until things had improved, and at last, things had.

It's two-thirty a.m. – seven hours since I've been wheeled back into my room from Recovery. I'm wide awake and feel so excited I know that any more sleep will be impossible for a while yet. I carefully lift the front of the hospital gown away from my neck and gaze down at the tight bandages wrapped round my chest. Even with all this padding, the effect is instant; instead of the 'terrible twins' examining the floor (as they seem to have done their entire life) they're now taking an interest in their surroundings, and examining the rather boring painting on the wall opposite the bed!

After about half an hour of navel gazing (will this novelty never wear off?) I reach for the television remote and flick through those God-awful infomercials. Wow, a steam mop that can be used on a timber floor or carpet or tiles and then have the ability to 'de-crease' your favourite outfit. Yeah, well I've just had my new favourite outfit 'decreased' several hours ago, so you can stick your magic mop!

I trawl through the television stations and finally hear some 'easy listening' 60s music. How simple was life back then as I coasted through my teenage years. Each weekend, Jan and Dean took me to Surf City (that's if I wasn't going 'Downtown' with Petula) and Manfred Mann's 'Do Wah Diddy' made perfect sense.

It was a long wait to be taken into theatre today – a long and hungry one.

'Don't have anything to eat or drink after six a.m. and be here by eleven a.m.,' they instructed.

I slept in, so was shovelling food down my throat at five fifty-eight a.m. Needn't have worried, as I didn't get into theatre till four p.m.

It's not always good to have this amount of time to think because one story, in particular, kept running around my head. A few years ago I was picking up my meds from the pharmacy when I noticed a new chemist was filling in for my regular.

As he handed over the filled scrips, he told me his mother had been through breast cancer a few years ago. 'One piece of advice I'd give you is this,' he said. 'Don't be tempted to go in for breast reconstruction afterwards.'

I was puzzled as to why he felt the need to give any advice to a total stranger, let alone something so personal, but he hadn't finished.

'Soon after the operation, she developed secondary cancer and I think it was opening her up again that did it!'

I wasn't surprised to see that he didn't last long at the pharmacy.

My surgeon is in very early the next morning and eases the bandages away so he can check his handiwork. 'Hope I haven't made them too small,' he says.

The man's joking, of course – could there be such an animal?

I take yet another opportunity to admire his handiwork and notice that although they're now the same size, the lack of a nipple on the left makes them fraternal not identical twins. The doctor had told me I could have a nipple tattooed on further down the track, but then I found out that a dolphin probably wouldn't be an option, so I may not go ahead. Come to think of it, I could have a small feline instead. This would be in memory of the cat's arse look I carried round for the last few years due to some very creative surgery with my partial mastectomy!

It's now mid-morning of the next day and I'm waiting for morning tea. (Note to self: don't eat your way back to a double-F cup!)

Suddenly a woman's face appears from around the curtain. 'Hello, gorgeous girl. I was checking the patient list and saw your name. What are you doing here?' she said.

I held my arms out as my wonderful breast care nurse wrapped me in a warm hug. 'Oh, Jane, how great to see you,' I said. 'You're just in time to check out the new puppies!'

I've spoken before of these very special BCNs (yes, I still call them boobs, chests and norks) and in my case, I had won the lottery with my very special nurse. She sat on the end of the bed and we caught up on each other's news over the past few years. I was shocked to hear she'd had a dreadful health scare with her husband recently but, knowing the dedication she has to her work, I bet her patients were still looked after in her gentle, caring manner.

'I can't believe it, Jane,' I said, smiling at my angel. 'You were there to wipe my tears on the day of diagnosis and now you're here to witness the final step. I couldn't have written a better ending!'

www.ingramcontent.com/pod-product-compliance
Ingram Content Group UK Ltd.
Pitfield, Milton Keynes, MK11 3LW, UK
UKHW041950230426
12048UKWH00008B/254